THE STOPLIGHT DIET
FOR CHILDREN

THE STOPLIGHT DIET
FOR CHILDREN

An Eight-Week Program for
Parents and Children

LEONARD H. EPSTEIN, Ph.D.,
and SALLY SQUIRES, M.S.

FOREWORD BY JANE E. BRODY

LITTLE, BROWN AND COMPANY
Boston   Toronto

FIRST EDITION

This work was developed under a grant from the U.S. Public
Health Service, National Institute of Child Health and Human
Development. However, the content does not necessarily reflect
the position or policy of that agency, and no official endorsement
of these materials should be inferred.

For reasons of privacy, the names of diet participants who are
discussed in this book have been changed.

Library of Congress Cataloging-in-Publication Data
Epstein, Leonard H.
   The stoplight diet for children.

   1. Obesity in children.   2. Reducing diets.
3. Children—Nutrition.   I. Squires, Sally.   II. Title.
[DNLM: 1. Child Nutrition—popular works.   2. Diet,
Reducing—in infancy & childhood.   WD 212 E64s]
RJ399.C6E67   1988   613.2'5'088054   86-34283
ISBN 0-316-24575-5

10 9 8 7 6 5 4 3 2 1
RRD-VA
Designed by Patricia Girvin Dunbar

*Published simultaneously in Canada
by Little, Brown & Company (Canada) Limited*

PRINTED IN THE UNITED STATES OF AMERICA

To my father and mother — L.H.E.

*To John, Eric, and Ian (and L.B.) for their love,
support, and help* — S.S.

Contents

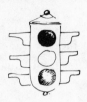

Acknowledgments

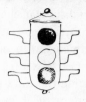

Books are always the end product of a collaborative effort by many people, and this one is no exception. The work of many dedicated individuals, from the laboratory to the editorial offices, went into the production of this book.

The Stoplight Diet for Children would never have been possible without the participation of the 1,000 family members who have enrolled in our program at the University of Pittsburgh School of Medicine during the past decade. For their time, dedication, commitment, and courage, we will always be immensely grateful.

Research support for the Childhood Obesity program, which grew into the Stoplight Diet for Children, came from the National Institute of Child Health and Human Development. Without this help, neither the program nor the book would have been possible.

Numerous people at the University of Pittsburgh School of Medicine have also made major contributions to this project. Dr. Rena Wing, a psychologist at the University of Pittsburgh, served as a consultant in designing the research during all stages of development of our program. Project nutritionist Alice Valoski, M.S., R.N., created a substantial portion of the treatment materials used in our Pittsburgh program. She also refined the diet and performed nutrient analyses. Others who have contributed to the design and implementation of our program over the past decade include Frank Andrasik, Steven Beck, Barbara Dickson, Randi Koeske, Mary Jean Kress, Margaret Nuss, Deborah Ossip-Klein, Barbara Penner, Linda Steranchek, Camille Szparaga, Karen Woodall, and John Zidansek. Pat Cluss made important contributions to our understanding of the role parents play in helping children to lose weight. In addition, Dorothy Becker and Lew Kuller helped to extend the scope of our research to include heart disease in children, while Bob Robertson lent his expertise in exercise physiology, and secretary Bea Tombosky spent many hours typing treatment protocols and food guides.

Thanks goes as well to former *Washington Post* editors Ben Cason and Carol Krucoff for producing the kind of flexible newsroom environment that enables a full-time medical reporter to write a book in her off hours.

Special recognition goes to John Wilhelm for the many hours he spent reading drafts of the manuscript and for offering numerous thoughtful suggestions for revision. Without his support and encouragement, this book would never have been possible.

Finally, we offer special thanks to Senior Editor Fredrica S. Friedman, her assistant Lori Goldstein, and copy editor Michael Brandon, who carefully shepherded this book through the editing and publication process. Their thoughtful suggestions and attention to detail are very much appreciated.

Foreword

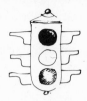

Once upon a time, not all that long ago, parents wanted their children to be fat, or at least pleasingly plump. In the days before antibiotics, immunizations, and a dependable food supply, those extra pounds were a survival advantage. As recently as the 1940s and 1950s, parents and grandparents anxiously poured thick shakes down the throats of reluctant young eaters to fatten them up. My own grandmother, frightened by my pencil-thin grade-school body, regularly plied me with sticks of butter, slabs of cheese, whole cans of evaporated milk, and an unlimited amount of ice cream.

Now as I struggle with the threat of middle-aged spread, those fat-rich orgies are but a vague, ironic memory. And for many who will become middle-aged in the twenty-first century, even the memory will not exist. Today's parents are clearly antifat — in their diets, and in their own and their children's bodies. The lean, sinewy look is in and is likely to remain fashionable throughout our lifetimes. Children who are not threatened by devastating infections and periodic famines are clearly better off without the burden of excess bodily baggage.

Let's face it: It's just no fun being a fat kid. Not only must a fat child suffer the slings and arrows of outrageous epithets (Fatso, Blimp, Blob, Slob — often used by shameless peers in place of the child's given name), but signs of frank discrimination can show up as early as age three or four. When preschool children are asked to choose friends and teammates, heavier children are among the last to be selected. Overweight children have a harder time keeping up with their pals. They don't run as fast or climb as agilely. They can't wear all the in fashions. In some places, they simply don't fit — literally.

But while the social pain is most apparent, the price that being overweight exacts on physical health can be even worse. Fat children are more likely to develop dangerously elevated blood pressure, even before they enter high school. Their coronary arteries may accumulate more fatty deposits, increasing their risk of a premature heart attack. As they get older, they are more susceptible to diabetes and arthritis.

The time to help a child who has a weight problem is now, while he or she is still a child. The longer you wait, the harder the task becomes and the more emotional scars the child accumulates meanwhile. It is not safe to assume the child will outgrow his or her "baby fat." Many never do, at least not without a special effort. And those who are still overweight as adolescence yields to young adulthood can look forward to a lifelong struggle against overabundant fat cells that seem determined to stay filled.

There are three main periods in a child's life when the number of body cells where fat is stored increases rapidly: before birth, during infancy, and during early adolescence. Fat cells, once formed, become permanent body residents. They can get fatter or thinner, but they won't disappear. A child who is still fat by mid- to late adolescence is destined to be burdened by excess fat cells for his or her entire life. Without intervention, three-fourths of fat teens will be fat adults.

What can you, the parent of an overweight child, do to help? First, you must resist all temptation to control your child's food intake through ridicule, deprivation, fad diets, formulas, fasting, pills, potions, and similar unhealthy tactics. Many young lives have been ruined by such extreme measures. Besides, severe caloric restriction in a child can result in impaired growth. Rather, the goal should be to teach your children how to live normally with food: how to eat regular meals and wholesome snacks, how to choose foods that are rich in nutrients but relatively low in calories, and how to save those very tempting, high-calorie, low-nutrient no-nos as treats for special occasions. Equally important is how your children expend the calories they consume. It's time to turn this country of young "couch potatoes" into lively sprouts. Television and motorized transportation have wreaked havoc on the physical fitness of the nation's youth. It is not only easier, it is also safer to limit a child's girth through physical exercise rather than stringent dieting.

The Stoplight Diet for Children gives you a near-perfect method for realizing these goals. Though I wish *diet* would be dropped from the dictionary, the program described in this book is not a diet in the strict sense of the word. It's a game plan. No child is told what to eat and when. Rather, the child and his or her entire family learn about foods and their relative nutrient and caloric values. The various types of foods are categorized according to the colors of a stoplight: green for the all-you-can-eat foods, yellow for the foods that are nutritionally desirable but calorically on the heavy side, and red for the foods that are calorically overloaded, whether or not they are nutritionally defensible. Confronted with a "red" food, a child need not turn away, but merely stop and think: Do I really want this? Do I want all of it? How many other red foods have I had this week?

The family also learns about "life-style exercise" — the kinds of regular physical activities that we all can pursue in the course of our daily routine. You need not become a "jock" to benefit; in fact, the program suggests starting with just 50 extra calories a day expended through physical activity.

A plan like this requires parental participation. It would hardly do to serve everyone but the fat child an ice-cream sundae for dessert, or to let everyone else in the house nibble on chips and cookies while watching television but insist that the fat child eat only at the table and only at mealtime. Even if other members of the family do not have a weight problem, the principles of the Stoplight Diet can promote healthful eating and exercise habits — the kinds of habits that can help to ward off the chronic, disabling diseases that now tarnish the golden years of so many senior citizens.

There is another good thing about the Stoplight Diet: it insists that the child is ultimately responsible for making it work. And it provides an enjoyable and educational series of tasks to help motivate the child and keep him or her on track week after week. It is not a diet your child — or you, for that matter — will ever have to abandon. Because it is not just a diet. It's an eating and exercise management plan that everyone in the family can adopt and use indefinitely, for better health and a better life.

— JANE E. BRODY
New York Times Personal Health columnist

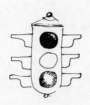

Part One

PARENTS' GUIDE
TO THE
STOPLIGHT DIET
FOR CHILDREN

Why the
Stoplight Diet
Is Right for
Your Family

The number of American children who weigh too much has reached epidemic proportions. It is estimated that as many as four million children between the ages of six and eleven risk serious health problems because of excess weight. In a nationwide study of more than 7,000 children, Dr. William Dietz of the New England Medical Center in Boston estimated that one in five American children is obese. (Children who weigh a minimum of 20 percent more than the national average for someone their age, height, and sex are considered obese; those who are at least 10 percent above their ideal weight but under 20 percent over it are considered overweight.)

Until recently, few parents knew what to do for their overweight or obese children. Diets for children simply were not available. Some parents, afraid that they might stunt their child's growth, were reluctant even to try to help their fat son or daughter lose weight. Others tried and failed. They found that they could not keep Susie or Scott from raiding the cookie jar, munching on potato chips, or drinking sugary soda pop when these foods were available for other family members.

The Stoplight Diet for Children can change all that. What you will read here can help you improve your children's lives permanently. They will feel better and be healthier. And so will you.

The Stoplight Diet for Children is a scientifically proved program based on a decade of our research at the Western Psychiatric Institute and Clinic, University of Pittsburgh School of Medicine. By following what we will teach you here, you will join the growing ranks of over

250 families — more than 1,000 people — who have already completed the program.

While the Stoplight Diet is specially designed for children six through twelve years old, parents and teenaged siblings can reap the rewards too. One mother who participated in our program used the Stoplight Diet to break a three-generation chain of obesity in her family. Mary Ann Lucci had struggled with being overweight since she was a teenager. Her mother and aunts are also obese, and for thirty-five years, Mary Ann had tried numerous diets to keep off weight without success. It was not until her two daughters, ten-year-old Lena and six-year-old Anna were each 25 pounds overweight that she decided to find some way to halt the cycle once and for all. "I just didn't want them to go through what had happened to me as a fat teenager," Mary Ann explained. Together with her husband, Frank, the family embarked on the Stoplight Diet and lost a combined total of 140 pounds. Today, two years later, they still maintain their slim new figures.

You can help your family lose weight too. We are going to show you how. Our knowledge comes from years of scientific research on the Stoplight Diet — much of it funded by the federal government through the National Institute of Child Health and Human Development. Our studies show one result again and again: The Stoplight Diet works. Your children will lose weight and — most important — will keep it off. Ours is a clinically proved program that works not just during a few months of dieting but over the long term.

We also want you to know that the Stoplight program is not just a diet; it is designed to change your children's eating habits and health behavior for good. By teaching them about nutrition and exercise, it gives them important new skills that will serve them for the rest of their lives, regardless of whether they need to lose 10 pounds, 20 pounds, or nothing at all.

Because this is a family-based program, it will help everyone in your family — children, teenagers, and adults, regardless of weight — to maintain a balanced but low-fat diet through good food choices and sensible portion sizes — precisely the kind of nutritional philosophy recently advocated by such prestigious organizations as the National Cancer Institute, the American Heart Association, the National Academy of Sciences, and the American Academy of Pediatrics.

As recently as September of 1986, the American Academy of Pediatrics Committee on Nutrition advised its members on a prudent dietary life-style for children: "Counseling on the maintenance of ideal body weight and a regular exercise program . . . should be a routine part of all health supervision visits." In addition, the committee suggested that "detection of obesity [in children] by measuring height and weight . . . according to the schedules published by the Academy will permit the early recognition and treatment of obesity and hypertension [high blood pressure]."

The Stoplight Diet takes time, dedication, and work. The pounds will not magically "melt away" overnight; instead, your children will lose weight steadily and safely. Our program operates on the belief that a gradual weight loss, one that takes off about 1 pound per week, is by far the best route to permanent success.

The Stoplight Diet reduces calories to the safest minimum level that will provide adequate nutrition for good health and development in growing children while still guaranteeing weight loss. Because the diet emphasizes low-calorie, low-fat, but healthful foods — skim milk, fruits and vegetables, whole grains, poultry, fish, and lean meats — children find that they can lose weight and not feel hungry. And since there are no "forbidden" foods, they never have to feel deprived.

There is no rigid menu to follow in the Stoplight Diet. This is a program designed to be tailored to your overweight child's — and your family's — needs and tastes. You are in control here. Calorie counting is important, but it is not the primary focus. Instead, the emphasis is on making smart food choices and paying attention to portion sizes.

All food on the Stoplight Diet is divided into three simple, color-coded categories: red, yellow, and green — just like the signals on a traffic light. Children find this concept appealing and easy to learn. Following the Stoplight signals makes dieting fun and almost a game for them.

The Stoplight Diet appeals psychologically to children for several reasons. Unlike other programs, it involves the entire family. All of you will work together to help the overweight children in your household lose weight. This approach gives them much-needed moral support. The Stoplight Diet also places no blame about who is responsible for a child being fat. We start with the premise that no one is at fault — neither child nor parent. Rather, it is important simply to move ahead and help your child lose weight.

In our program at the University of Pittsburgh, children also learn that they are not alone in their battle against obesity. Your children will learn that same lesson through the special chapters that have been written expressly for them — another unique feature of the Stoplight Diet. Each week, your children will read about other children who faced the same challenges — and triumphs — that they will face during the Stoplight Diet.

People lose weight most successfully when they diet with a partner. Research shows that weight-loss programs that focus only on one person in a family simply do not work in the long run. If you have ever tried putting your son or daughter on a diet while the rest of the family indulges in such "regular" food as fried chicken, french fries, cookies, ice cream, and cake, you already know what we mean.

The Stoplight Diet works in part because it relies on teamwork. You or your spouse will be your child's diet partner, and we will be cheering you on. Your participation and that of your whole family is important for your child's success. Even if you do not need to lose weight yourself, you can still reap the rewards of better nutrition: More fruits and vegetables. More complex carbohydrates. Less fat. Plus, you will learn about exercise and about how to fit it into a busy schedule.

Our experience with overweight children has shown that they want to lose weight. They do not like being the brunt of jokes or teasing because of their weight. Nor do they enjoy such nicknames as Fatso or Tubby. Like adults, overweight children often do not know how to lose weight or how to keep it off. They frequently hide their feelings about being overweight from their parents. One ten-year-old boy happily confessed to his parents after losing 11 pounds on the Stoplight Diet: "This summer I'm going to wear shorts again. Last year, I didn't want to because my legs were too fat."

As you read this book you will see how the Stoplight Diet has changed the lives of the children and parents who tested it at the University of Pittsburgh. We hope their success stories will encourage you to apply the principles of the Stoplight Diet to your own situation. Perhaps you and your family will be like the Fosters, who learned how to "overcome thirty years of bad eating habits." Or maybe you will find inspiration from the restaurant-owning Solomons who followed the Stoplight Diet despite eating many dinners away from home.

Most important, you can now give your children a gift that will change their lives forever. Not only can you help them put the brakes on obesity, but you offer them a green light to a lifetime of good eating and exercise habits. In all likelihood, you will help prolong their lives.

Your children will appreciate your help and support in losing weight. After eleven-year-old Melissa went on the Stoplight Diet — and stayed slim for more than a year — she said: "Mom, I'm really glad you are my mother. I'm really glad that you put me on the Stoplight Diet."

Stop, Look, and Listen

Sandra Solomon and her husband, Jason, are both in their early thirties. Neither they nor their eight-year-old son, Oliver, has ever had a weight problem, so they were at a loss about how to help their eleven-year-old daughter, Julie.

"Ever since she was a baby, Julie loved to eat," Sandra says. "My husband owns several restaurants, where we frequently eat, and Julie always loved the variety of foods. She could eat adult portions at ages when other children were just learning about 'grown-up' food."

As Julie's appetite continued to grow, so did her waist — and her thighs, her hips, and her stomach. By the time she was eight years old, "she was a real butterball," Sandra says. Shopping for clothes became an arduous task, one that began hopefully in department stores and ended with discouragement — and sometimes tears — in small, depressing shops for chubby girls.

At home, Sandra talked to Julie about dieting and looked for ways to help her lose weight. "We tried cutting out desserts for a while," Sandra says. "Then I made special meals for Julie, but that was difficult and no fun for anyone. There was tension in the air as we all ate a regular dinner and Julie ate her diet meal. I'm sure she felt deprived, and I felt guilty for eating other things in front of her."

While watching television one night, Sandra and her husband saw a public-service announcement about a research program for overweight children at the University of Pittsburgh. They jotted down the name and phone number and called the next day. Julie had an appointment within a week.

The family spent the next several months learning how to alter their eating habits to help Julie lose weight on the Stoplight Diet. Fattening "red foods" were banned from the house the first week, and still have not found their way back into the Solomons' kitchen over the past three years.

Today, Julie is a trim, soft-spoken preteen. "The days of being fat are over for me," says Julie, with a shy smile and a quick glance to her mother for reassurance as she describes the metamorphosis she underwent.

Like most overweight children, Julie often found herself the brunt of cruel teasing from classmates. The jokes and taunts only served to further undermine her already poor self-image.

"I just wanted to be like everyone else," Julie says. On the Stoplight

Diet, that wish became a reality. Over six months, Julie lost 12 pounds. She exercises now, and has even taken up ice skating. But more important, she has stayed slim for the past three years. Her family has also benefited — not just from seeing Julie look better and feel better about herself, but also from learning improved eating habits that continue to serve them well.

"My husband, who has always been a little too thin, now eats better than he ever has," Sandra says. "The focus is different for us now, and I wouldn't have it any other way."

"I wouldn't either," Julie says with a big grin.

If you are like most parents, the realization that your child is overweight was probably as emotional as Mrs. Solomon's. You may have felt angry; frightened; worried. And you probably felt helpless.

Jerry King, a forty-two-year-old divorced father of two boys, aged eight and twelve, recalls those feelings. He had thought his children looked a bit heavy on their weekend visits, and had even encouraged them to cut back on the junk food they enjoyed eating so much. But it was not until he took them shopping for new trousers and sports jackets that he realized how bad the situation had become. "The saleslady just stood there, with the tape measure dangling around her neck," Jerry says. "She shook her head and said, 'I'm sorry, sir, but we just can't help you. We don't carry anything that could fit them.' She suggested we try a store in the next town that specialized in clothing for chubby kids. My oldest son was embarrassed. My youngest son clung to me in tears and wailed about not wanting to go shopping anymore. It was one of the worst days I've ever had."

For other parents, the realization that their children need to lose weight may crystallize in an emotional scene after school. "They called me Fatso," sniffed six-year-old Catherine Walker to her mother after painful teasing at the school playground. For Mike Charles, age nine, the taunts came during Saturday-morning soccer practice, as he waddled down the field, puffing to keep up with his teammates. "I don't want to go back there," he solemnly told his father. "They laughed at me and called me fat."

"When he told me about that," says Mike's father, "I felt like someone had ripped my heart out. I knew that we had a problem. I just couldn't deny it any longer, but until then I kept thinking that he'd grow out of it."

Some parents overhear teasing between siblings, or realize that it is not "just baby fat" the pediatrician is talking about when she tells you that your child's body weight does not match the normal-growth charts that are based on height, sex, and age.

The first step if you suspect a weight problem is to measure your child's height in inches with a tape measure. Then weigh your son or daughter (in pounds), preferably in the morning, before breakfast. For the most accurate measurement of body weight, it is best for your child to be undressed or wearing only underwear during the weigh-in.

Compare your child's measurements with those in the ideal-weight tables in appendix A, which have been calculated from heights and weights in the general population. The measurements listed tell you what the average weight is for children of the same height, age, and sex. These figures in themselves do not diagnose obesity (for instance, they might not apply to a child with a large frame), but they are a good first check. They will also help pinpoint a developing weight problem.

As mentioned earlier, children who are under 20 percent above the ideal weight for someone their height, age, and sex but at least 10 percent over the ideal are considered overweight. Children who weigh 20 percent or more above the ideal are defined as obese. For example, say your eleven-year-old son is 60 inches tall. His ideal weight is 90 pounds, as shown in the appendix A table for boys. Since he weighs 104 pounds, he is thus 14 pounds heavier than the ideal weight for a boy in his height and age group. That works out to about 16 percent more than his ideal weight (14 divided by 90 equals 0.155, or 16 percent). In this case, your son is overweight and needs the Stoplight Diet. If your son weighs 98 pounds, he is a little heavier than ideal but does not qualify as being overweight since he is within 10 percent of the norm. We do not recommend the full Stoplight Diet program for children who are just a few pounds heavier than average. They certainly can benefit from learning the lessons included here about nutrition and exercise, but we do not think that their weight warrants having them go through the full eight-week program.

On the other hand, if your eleven-year-old son weighs 109 pounds, he is more than 20 percent above the ideal weight and qualifies as obese. In this case, you should use the full Stoplight Diet program to help him slim down. Should your son or daughter weigh 50 percent or more above the weight considered ideal — and we have seen children in the Stoplight Diet program who are this seriously obese — you should seek help beyond this book. Consult your family physician, pediatrician, or a local medical school or university that specializes in treating severe obesity. We recommend that you do this right away.

Another way to gauge your child's weight problem is to take a good, hard look at how his or her build compares with that of friends, classmates, and siblings. Is your son or daughter the largest child in the class? Does he or she dwarf other children the same age? How does one child in your family compare with another? (In Jerry King's family, the youngest son, David, had the same size waist as his older brother, Sid, who was four years older and more than a head taller.)

Also look at clothes. One mother whose child successfully mastered the Stoplight Diet says that she can spot overweight kids just by their pant legs. "The hems are easily six to ten inches deep because the child needs such a large-size waist, but usually his or her legs have not grown," she says.

The ideal weight you find in appendix A, give or take 10 percent, is your child's weight-loss goal for now. Update this "goal weight" every six months — or whenever a visible change in height occurs. As children grow taller, their ideal weight needs to be recalculated and their goal weight adjusted to allow for their increase in height.

As you gauge the weight of your son or daughter, don't forget to check your weight and that of your spouse. Compare the results with the figures listed in the ideal-weight table for adults in appendix A. What you weigh is important. Studies show that overweight parents tend to increase the chance that their children will be too heavy.

TIPS ON WEIGHING IN

• Find your child's ideal weight using the tables in appendix A. (For your child's age, round to the nearest year. For height, round to the nearest inch.)

• Calculate the extent of your child's weight problem: Subtract the child's ideal weight from the actual weight; then divide the result by the ideal weight and multiply by 100. This will give you the excess weight as a percentage of the ideal.

• Compare your child's height and weight with that of his or her classmates and friends the same age, and be alert for additional clues, such as a much older sibling who is the same size.

• Check with your pediatrician or family doctor. A physician can help you set a goal weight for your child to attain if he or

continued on next page

she is overweight. In most cases, the goal weight will be within 10 percent of the ideal weight given in appendix A. This goal-weight will need to be updated periodically as your child grows older and taller.

• Measure your own weight and that of your spouse. Then check the ideal-weight table for adults in appendix A to see where you fit. Children with overweight parents run an added risk of being heavy and even obese, particularly if these children put on extra pounds in childhood.

If your child's actual weight is less than 10 percent over the ideal weight, dieting is not necessary. Your child is within the acceptable range. You may still use the information in the Stoplight Diet to teach your child about better nutrition and exercise, but do not limit calories for weight loss.

If your child is at least 10 percent above the ideal weight, but less than 20 percent over it he or she is overweight but not obese. In this case, you can use the Stoplight Diet to help trim pounds. But be sure to monitor weight loss very carefully, because your child may quickly reach the ideal-weight range in a few weeks, and then will need to go on a maintenance program (as described in Week 8 of the Stoplight Diet).

If your child weighs 20 percent or more above the ideal weight, he or she is obese. The Stoplight Diet can help you guide such a child through a safe and healthy weight-loss program while you both learn about better nutrition and exercise.

If your child's weight exceeds the ideal by 50 percent or more, immediately consult a physician for help or contact a university-based program specializing in obesity.

The Health Effects of Obesity

Children pay both an emotional and physical price when they weigh too much. At the best of moments, obese children are called "pleasingly plump." It is said in polite, hushed tones that they have not yet outgrown their "baby fat." But then there are the times when they are teased by classmates and are chided for their added weight. They earn nicknames like Fat Albert and Thunder Thighs — labels that leave the psyche smarting long into adulthood. It is no wonder then, that these children may suffer from low self-esteem and a poor body image. "Obesity creates an enormous psychological burden," a special National Institutes of Health panel concluded during a 1985 conference. "In fact, in terms of suffering, this burden may be the greatest adverse effect of obesity."

For overweight children, the psychological suffering often translates to behavior problems: trouble in school, shyness, hyperactivity, social withdrawal, or depression. Most of these children are not clinically depressed; they just feel "down," left out, and usually without friends. Repeated teasing by unthinking classmates leaves them emotionally bruised and wary of other children. They tend to find solace playing quietly in their rooms, or escape by watching television and by eating — activities that only make their condition worse.

Not only will the Stoplight Diet help heavy children lose weight and feel better about themselves, it will teach them about good nutrition and exercise, and will minimize the physical health hazards they face. As the National Institutes of Health noted in a February 1985 consensus statement, "the evidence is now overwhelming that obesity, defined as excessive storage of energy in the form of fat, has adverse effects on health and longevity." Too much weight in childhood helps lay the foundation for a host of serious illnesses later in life: cancer, heart disease, high blood pressure, stroke, kidney disease, and diabetes. The biggest killers in the United States today are linked to excess weight and poor nutrition.

Overweight children often have elevated levels of the blood fats known as cholesterol and triglycerides, some types of which cause hardening of the arteries (atherosclerosis) and lead to heart disease and premature death. (Fat is unable to move by itself through the blood, so the body packages it in bundles comprised of fat and protein, which then travel through the blood. Cholesterol and triglycerides are part of these packages.)

Our studies show that after two months of dieting, children on the Stoplight Diet have significantly lowered levels of blood cholesterol and triglycerides. The diet also helps them to increase the level of a protective type of cholesterol in their blood called high-density lipoprotein, or HDL. HDL is thought to help clear cholesterol from the blood and thus protect against clogged arteries.

All three changes — lower levels of total cholesterol and triglycerides, and higher levels of HDL — point to better health, particularly when it comes to decreasing the risk of heart disease.

Several major studies also have shown that many overweight children have high blood pressure. Even having a blood pressure reading in the upper quarter of the normal range — as overweight children often do — puts these children on "a collision course for [having] high blood pressure as adults," according to Dr. Jeremiah Stamler, an authority on blood pressure and cardiovascular disease at Northwestern University.

The Stoplight Diet is effective in lowering blood pressure. Six months after beginning the Stoplight Diet, obese children of heavy parents as well as those of thin parents show significant decreases in systolic blood pressure (the pressure when the heart contracts) and diastolic blood pressure (the pressure when the heart dilates and allows blood to rush into it).

The Stoplight Diet program is one of the first research efforts in the country designed to change children's eating and exercise behavior. It leads a new trend designed to catch children early, while there is still time to make these changes habits for a lifetime. The American Heart Association, Stanford University, and the American Academy of Pediatrics are among the growing number of organizations and institutions that advocate teaching children about safety, exercise, nutrition, and better health.

The National Institutes of Health also reported that it "views with concern the increasing frequency of obesity in children and adolescents. Obese children should be encouraged to stay within normal limits."

Who Is at Risk?

Almost a dozen scientific studies have examined the problem of obesity among the American children and teenagers. Their conclusion? That from 10 percent to 30 percent of Americans between eight to eighteen years old are obese. The most comprehensive of these research projects, mentioned earlier, found that one in every five American children between six to eleven years old is obese — which means that an estimated four million children battle an excess-weight problem by age eleven. If your child thinks that he is the only one who faces a weight problem, you should reassure him that this is not so.

Who is at greatest risk for obesity? The results of various studies paint an interesting picture of who these children are likely to be. For instance, children from small families are more prone to putting on unwanted pounds than are those from large families, and a child with no siblings faces about twice the chance of becoming heavy as does one with three brothers or sisters. Scientists do not know for certain why this should be true, but they theorize that an only child usually has unlimited access to food, unlike those from larger families, who must learn to share what they eat with brothers and sisters.

City children are more likely to be overweight than are children from the country. Obesity experts think that this is because the city offers less opportunity for exercise and more for eating. Urban children rarely have yards in which to play; their activities are likely to be confined to the indoors.

Children who live in colder climates — the Northeast and the Midwest — also run a higher risk of added pounds than do children who live in the South and the West. Experts believe this is largely because people lead more sedentary lives during inclement winter.

Family income also affects the risk of developing weight problems. Lower-income families are more likely to have children with excess-weight problems than are upper-income families, while middle-income families fall right between the other two. There are many possible reasons for these weight differences among children from different socioeconomic backgrounds. None of the reasons have been studied scientifically. The most widely held opinion is that more-affluent parents may be more attuned to the health problems of obesity and may try to help their children slim down earlier — and can afford experts who provide assistance.

But regardless of family size, geographic location, climate, or family income, the strongest indication of whether a child will be overweight is parent weight. Without help, the children at greatest risk of carrying unwanted pounds into adulthood are those whose mother or father — or both — are obese. As with many medical conditions, including diabetes and heart disease, it seems that at least some types of obesity have a familial component — that the tendency to be fat is handed down in some families the way that eye color, height, and curly hair are passed from generation to generation. For instance, the adorable but obese six-month-old infant whose mother or father is also obese has about five times the chance of becoming an obese adult as a normal-weight infant with normal-weight parents. Findings from a 1976 government-sponsored ten-state survey show that such a propensity for extra weight continues with age. By age twelve, children with an obese mother or father have, on average, three times more fat on their arms than comparable children with parents of normal weight.

One of the reasons why characteristics such as weight tend to cluster in families is genetics. Some of the most recent evidence illustrating the contribution of genetics to obesity comes from a study of Danish adults who were adopted as children. Conducted by Dr. Albert Stunkard of the University of Pennsylvania and published in 1986, the study compared the body weight of adoptees to that of their biological parents and that of their adopted parents. The conclusion: the body weight of adoptees much more closely matched the body weight of their biological parents, which points to the important role that genes may play in obesity.

Regardless of how a child becomes obese, one trend is clear: without help, he or she is likely to be shadowed by obesity throughout life. Numerous studies show that all too often today's overweight child is tomorrow's fat adult:

• At age six months, about one of every seven obese infants is destined to be a fat adult.
• By age seven years, about four of every ten obese children will become overweight adults.
• At ages ten through thirteen years, about seven of every ten overweight children can count on carrying their extra pounds with them into adulthood.

"Present-day concerns about obesity relate both to the social unacceptability and the health hazard," reports the American Academy of Pediatrics in its widely used *Pediatric Nutrition Handbook*. "The fact that childhood obesity may persist into the adult years makes the condition especially challenging to those caring for children."

How the Stoplight Diet Can Help

The good news is that the Stoplight Diet successfully helps children lose weight because it starts with parents. You will teach your children not only new ways of eating, but also new activities that will help them lose those added pounds. With your help and support, they will discover that being normal weight is within their grasp.

As they achieve these goals, the personalities of children on the Stoplight Diet often change. Our studies show a clear pattern of improved behavior when children lose weight. They become less withdrawn. They perform better in school and are less aggressive.

Some parents have even seen differences in how much their children sleep. "It seemed like my older daughter, Lena, never slept more than an hour a night when she was overweight," recalls Mary Ann Lucci, the mother of two children who have lost a total of 51 pounds on the Stoplight Diet. "But when Lena had been on the diet for a couple of weeks, she started to sleep through the night again."

Many children show more confidence and greater self-esteem. They frequently gain new respect from family, friends, and teachers for losing weight. Mary Ann's younger daughter, six-year-old Anna, had been shy and withdrawn before losing 25 pounds on the Stoplight Diet. "Her whole personality has changed since she lost the weight," Mary Ann says. "If you had met her last year, she wouldn't have talked to you."

"Last year, I had only about one friend and that was Eric, and now I have lots," explains wide-eyed, soft-spoken Anna Lucci, who looks as though she has always been the slender child she is today. As a reminder of how much her daughters have accomplished, Mary Ann Lucci carries school pictures in her wallet from the previous year and proudly shares her daughters' triumph. The photographs reveal two little girls with the same large, brown eyes and long, dark hair. But there the before-and-after resemblance ends. The pictures show two overtly obese children, who appear almost as round as they are tall. Anna is clearly uncomfortable in the picture, a sullen-looking, unhappy child, far different from how she appears today.

Although she is still very young, Anna knows that the weight loss and how she feels about losing those pounds are responsible for the changes in her life. The lost pounds have revealed a new Anna — one who is happier and far more outgoing, one who enjoys being with people in ways she never did before.

"I didn't get invited to any parties last year," confesses Anna as she plays with a strand of her long, brown hair in the coy yet slightly self-conscious manner of a six-year-old. "Now I've been invited to about ten parties this year already."

Even her young friends recognize changes in Anna. "My friend Katie, she came up to me and said, 'I like you better because now you aren't fat anymore,' " Anna says, flashing a shy smile.

The children who have benefited from the Stoplight Diet also like themselves better. They are proud of their new figures. "Now we catch our son admiring his body in the mirror," explained the mother of one fifth-grade boy who trimmed 11 pounds. "He's taken an interest in clothes. He's much more outgoing and confident."

The children themselves see differences in their abilities. Without those extra pounds they find new energy and their physical fitness increases. "I can run faster," says Anna Lucci's older sister, Lena, who lost 26 pounds on the Stoplight Diet. "Now I can beat some people that I couldn't beat before."

Lena has also improved in another favorite sport — softball. "Last year, I was so fat I couldn't even hit the ball," says Lena, an outgoing ten-year-old who is now trim and long-legged. This year she is not only hitting the ball but also running around the bases with unprecedented speed.

Other children on the Stoplight Diet have taken up gymnastics, ballet, and karate. Several girls have tried out and won coveted slots as cheerleaders and pom-pom girls.

But the best reward is how the children themselves feel. As one twelve-year-old graduate of the Stoplight Diet told her mother, "I know that I'll never be overweight again, and if I do start to gain weight, I know how to control it. I'm so glad that you helped me."

And parents who participate in the Stoplight Diet also benefit. At age thirty-five, Mary Ann Lucci went from a dress size 22 to a size 11 after she started the Stoplight Diet. Now normal weight for her height and age, Mary Ann had tried numerous other diets. In fact, she says, "My whole life has been a diet. Before, when I went on a diet, I would have quit by now. I always wanted it for myself, but I was never able to do it before. Now I can. And more importantly, so can my children."

How to Use This Book

It is best if you and your spouse read this entire book, so you understand the general concepts. Then go back and work through the program, week by week, with your children.

When you begin the Stoplight program, you will read one chapter a week in the Parents' Guide, part one of this book. Children will read the companion chapter in part two, written especially for them. You should also read the children's chapter as well, so you will know exactly what they are being taught and can better answer their questions.

In the weekly chapters, you will learn about nutrition, about how to support behavioral change in your children, and about how to record what you eat, how much you weigh, and the amount you exercise. You will learn about setting goals for your children and yourself.

At the end of most parents' chapters, there is a self-scored quiz. Some questions will cover what you have just read, while others will recap or embellish earlier information. It is important to take each quiz and measure what you have learned before reading further. This gives you the opportunity to pinpoint any questions you may have about the program, and offers you the chance to steadily increase your understanding and to review what might not be clear before you help your children learn the same information. You are about to become an expert — and a partner in your children's road to better health. We will be right at your side, guiding and cheering you on.

Once your children have read their weekly chapter, they too will be quizzed on the material they have learned. You can photocopy the quizzes and give each of your children a copy so that everyone can participate without marking in this book. But instead of having them score their own quizzes, you will help your children review their answers and thus target areas they might not have understood.

In the Stoplight Diet program we conduct at the University of Pittsburgh, parents and children meet weekly to discuss their progress. We cannot reproduce those weekly meetings for you, but we can offer some advice from parents like you who have participated in the program. As you read through this book, you will meet some of these parents and learn how they felt as they helped their children lose weight. We think you will benefit from their insight: how they felt, what parts of the program were easy to do, which areas were more difficult. You will have a chance to share their camaraderie, their laughter, and their tips for making the program the most successful possible.

While the Stoplight Diet is organized into eight weekly lessons, the lessons you learn here are geared toward maintaining weight loss not just for a few weeks, or a few months, but for the many years your children have ahead. Life goes on regardless of when your family chooses to diet. There are birthday celebrations, anniversaries, holidays, and family reunions. Can you imagine never eating ice cream again? Or cake? Or a candy bar? Few children or adults could adhere to a lifelong program like that.

The philosophy behind the Stoplight Diet program is that you do not have to force your children to make huge sacrifices during the recommended eight weeks of weight loss, or beyond, to maintain that weight loss for a lifetime. Diet martyrs rarely achieve their goals. We are going to teach you how everyone can have his cake and eat it too. But we also will not fool you: neither your children nor you can eat these foods limitlessly and still lose weight. Your goal is to control the food you consume and stop letting the food control you and your children.

Week 1
Learning and Teaching the Stoplight Signals

To lose weight, you and your children will learn how to classify foods by three main categories. The system is simple enough for children to understand and is easy to remember. Foods are grouped according to the colors of an ordinary traffic stoplight: red, yellow, and green. We have found that children as young as three years of age quickly catch on to the color-signal concept. Here is how it works:

Green foods on the Stoplight Diet are those that are very low in calories; you will encourage your sons and daughters to eat just about as many of these foods as they want. A food's actual color does not necessarily correspond to its food group color on the Stoplight Diet. Carrots are a green food. So are asparagus, lettuce, broccoli, tomatoes, and many other low-calorie vegetables. Such foods and beverages as coffee, tea, spices, herbs, and diet soda also count as green foods. In addition to being low in calories, most of the green foods are high in vitamins and minerals, high in fiber, and very low in fat — in other words, very nutritious.

Yellow foods, the mainstay of the Stoplight Diet, are those that are moderate in calories. This group includes most of the sources of protein, grains, milk and dairy foods, as well as fruits and vegetables. Yellow foods are essential for a well-balanced diet. They are rich in nutrients for the number of calories they provide, yet are low in fat. They help provide fiber and complex carbohydrates, vitamins and minerals, and the calories needed for energy. But they need to be eaten in moderation — and with caution — because overeating them results in so many calories being taken in that it is impossible to lose weight.

Red foods, on the other hand, generally provide very little nutrition for the amount of calories they carry. Among these are most high-calorie foods, fried foods, and the numerous diet foods patterned after high-calorie treats — for instance, diet candy, cookies, and ice cream. All alcoholic beverages are considered red.

Foods high in fat content are considered red: fried chicken, cream cheese, french fries, cream, whole milk, potato chips, ice cream, butter. Rich sauces are also red foods — mayonnaise, hollandaise, tartar sauce, hot fudge — because they are *calorie dense,* a term nutritionists use to describe foods that are high in calories (mainly fat) yet low in essential vitamins and minerals. Each gram of fat you eat contains roughly 9 calories — more than twice the number of calories contained in a gram of protein or in a gram of carbohydrates. (A gram is small — 28 grams make up an ounce.)

Other foods rate as red foods because they are particularly high in sugar, and low in other important nutrients. Jelly beans, marshmallows, peanut brittle, honey, cookies, cake, pie, Jell-O, and similar foods qualify for this reason.

Some foods that are high in nutrients are too calorie-dense to be ranked as a yellow food. Tuna packed in oil is one example of this type of red food. Others are bacon, duck, almonds, peanuts, and cashews.

To understand why such foods are classified as red foods, consider this partial breakdown of baked chicken and bologna:

Baked Chicken	*Bologna*
(about one breast)	(about one slice)
3-ounce portion (85.7 grams)	1.5-ounce portion (42.9 grams)
protein = 26.9 grams	protein = 5.4 grams
fat = 2.9 grams	fat = 12.6 grams
calories = 150	calories = 140
food group: yellow	food group: red

Choosing chicken over bologna means that you can consume about twice as much food for about the same number of calories. By eating chicken instead of bologna, you put yourself ahead of the game when it comes to choosing a lower-fat, higher-protein meal. The chicken has about 3 grams of fat — roughly one-fourth the amount of fat contained in the bologna. Put another way, only 27 calories in the chicken come from pure fat compared with a whopping 113 calories supplied by fat in the bologna.

In addition, the chicken contains more protein — 27 grams versus just 5 grams for the bologna. In calories, this is equivalent to 108 calories of protein for the chicken compared with only 22 calories of protein supplied by the bologna. All in all, the chicken is a much better nutritional choice, which is why baked chicken counts as a yellow food and bologna qualifies as a red food.

For a similar reason, deep-fried foods also turn on the red light. Eat a half cup of baked or broiled eggplant and you consume a mere 20 calories. But fry that same amount of eggplant — or any food, for that matter — and you may add up to 100 calories of fat per serving, with no additional nutrients. By limiting fried foods, you will also be meeting the recommendations of the American Heart Association and the National Cancer Institute to reduce total fat in the diet. Evidence suggests that high-fat diets increase your risk of heart disease and cancer, the two biggest killers in the United States.

Red foods also include many combination dishes — for example, certain casseroles, soups, sandwiches, and salads. By themselves, the individual ingredients may qualify as yellow or even green foods. But put them together and the calorie count soars and earns the food a ranking in the red category. Among these foods are lasagna, egg salad (made with mayonnaise), pot pies, and lobster Newburg.

We provide a complete listing of green, yellow, and red foods, including combination dishes, in appendix B, "The Stoplight Diet Food Guide." Since you will want to be creative and are likely to concoct new dishes that are not listed in the guide, we offer the following tips on determining whether a particular combination food ranks in the yellow or the red category:

If you use green foods, yellow foods, or both to prepare the dish and those ingredients contain a combined total of less than 350 calories per adult serving, then the combination dish qualifies as yellow food. But if the dish you are preparing contains a red food as an ingredient, or runs to 350 or more calories per adult serving, then it should be ranked as a red food. Remember that most combination dishes are served as the main dish for a meal.

As mentioned earlier, many so-called diet products have been assigned to the red-food category. Since these foods are generally low in calories, counting them as red foods may seem strange at first. But consider that they also contain few other nutrients. Many also earn the "diet" label only because they contain smaller portion sizes, not because they are special high-quality, low-calorie foods. And most important, since these diet products are eaten to imitate the consumption of other high-calorie foods, they do not help promote changes in eating habits, which is one of the major goals of the Stoplight Diet.

But, of course, there are exceptions. The rules of thumb in judging whether a diet food will be red, yellow, or green are as follows:

• Diet foods that imitate high-calorie foods are considered red. Examples are diet candy, diet cookies, diet ice cream, diet hot chocolate, and so forth.

• Diet foods that imitate a yellow food rank as yellow foods themselves. For instance, one slice of diet American cheese qualifies as a yellow food, because a slice of regular American cheese rates the same category.

• Diet beverages, on the other hand, fall into the green food group, but are not recommended in excessive amounts. Instead, we encourage ice water, fruit juice, or, for a carbonated beverage, a mixture of a few ounces of fruit juice with carbonated water.

• Low-calorie sugar substitutes such as NutraSweet may be consumed in soft drinks, but they are not allowed on foods. All other commercial diet products are considered red.

In general, *stop* when you see red foods, and support your children in doing the same. Temptation strikes everyone, fat or thin. Research at the University of Pittsburgh has shown that to be successful with the Stoplight Diet, you must not keep red foods in the home. When your children do eat red foods, limit the servings to four (or fewer) per week and make sure that they are consumed away from home: at school, at a restaurant, or at a party.

Of the twenty-one meals a child normally consumes each week, only five of them — usually weekday lunches — are regularly eaten away from home. By removing red foods from your house and limiting how many red foods your children can eat each week, you are helping them to gain control of their eating environment. The more control they have over their eating environment, the faster they will lose weight — and the better chance they have of keeping it off permanently.

You may find this change tough in the beginning. Many parents report that their children moan and complain about not having cake, ice cream, cookies, or other favorite red foods in the house. Ignore the complaints as much as you can. You are setting the rules. We will help by teaching your children why it is important for them not to eat red foods, but habits do not change overnight. As you go through the program, you will learn ways to praise and reinforce your children's new eating habits. But this will take some time.

Remember that red foods are not necessary to achieve a nutritionally balanced diet. And when you or your children do eat red foods, you must compensate to stay within the recommended daily calorie ranges you will learn about shortly. This means that red foods are eaten at the expense of other, more nutritious possibilities. So eat them with caution, and try to eat them infrequently, if at all.

Now that you know the signals of the Stoplight Diet, the next step is to teach your children about the red, yellow, and green food groups. Our studies show that most children quickly learn which foods fall into the various color categories by writing down what they eat during each meal and looking it up in "The Stoplight Diet Food Guide" (appendix B). We also recommend buying some inexpensive red, yellow, and green stickers. Place these on foods in your refrigerator and your cupboards. You can make a game out of it, by enlisting your children's help. When you go shopping, bring this book along. Have your children look up various foods as you place them in the shopping cart. They will learn fast — as will you — which foods fall into which category. Another recommendation: cut out pictures of food from old magazines and make a game out of having your children identify which foods are red, which are yellow, and which are green. In each of these learning exercises, be sure to have your children do the work. They will not learn the food signals if you do the work for them.

Calories

Scientific research has shown that the body needs a certain number of calories to fuel important, life-sustaining functions: breathing, digestion, keeping the heart beating, physical activity, and growth.

But too many calories means too much weight. To turn the tables and lose weight requires burning more calories than are eaten. You must burn off about 3,500 excess calories to lose a pound — or you must eat 3,500 calories less.

Based on various studies, the optimum calorie ranges listed at the top of page 25 have been set for adults and children who want to lose weight on the Stoplight Diet. Combined with additional guidelines for eating, which you will soon learn about, these calorie ranges will ensure a well-balanced diet capable of meeting the nutritional requirements for adults and for growing children. And by staying below the upper limits of these

RECOMMENDED CALORIE RANGES ON THE STOPLIGHT DIET

Participant	Number of Calories per day
Teenage and adult males	900 to 1,500
Teenage and adult females	900 to 1,200
Children, ages 8 to 12	900 to 1,200
Children, ages 6 and 7	1,000 to 1,200

calorie ranges you and your children can expect to lose weight gradually every week.

Members of the family who do not need to lose weight can still participate in the Stoplight Diet. To gauge how many calories are consumed each day, record what they eat for three days. During this time, they should eat normally; just measure and write down exactly what they consume. At the end of the three days, add the calories and divide the total by three for a daily average. This number should then be used as their optimum daily calorie count.

Limiting the amount of food eaten to 1,200 calories a day is *not* recommended for pregnant women, or for women who are nursing. For this or another medical condition — such as high blood pressure, heart disease, or diabetes — consult your doctor for further advice before beginning the Stoplight Diet.

Counting calories tells you how much is being eaten each day. Knowing which foods are red, yellow, and green is another nutritional guidepost. This enables you to choose more wisely what you and your children will eat. As a final check to make sure that your family is getting a nutritionally balanced diet, it is important that their food choices also meet the daily guidelines shown below, which are discussed more fully in Week 2.

BASIC FOUR FOOD GROUP SERVING GUIDELINES

Food Group	Number of Servings per Day
Protein (P)	2
Grains (G)	4
Fruits and vegetables (F&V)	4
Dairy (D)	3

Studies of children who have been on the Stoplight Diet show that they receive adequate amounts of vitamins and essential minerals. If you want to give your son or daughter one tablet daily of a children's multiple vitamin, feel free to do so. But avoid what vitamin experts call "overdosing" — giving more than 100 percent of the recommended daily allowance of any vitamin or mineral. More is not necessarily better when it comes to vitamins.

TIPS ON FOLLOWING THE STOPLIGHT DIET

- Stay within the daily recommended calorie range.
- Limit red foods to four or less per week.
- Remove all red foods from the house.
- Eat red foods only when away from home — for instance, at a party, at school, at a restaurant, or at a sports event.
- Eat three meals a day.
- Keep a good nutritional balance by eating the recommended number of servings daily from the Basic Four food groups.

Self-Monitoring

The Stoplight Diet is far more than a weight-loss program. It is also a very special tool designed to change health habits for good. By mastering this tool, you will reshape how your family eats and exercises.

One of the keys to changing habits is what psychologists call *self-monitoring*. There is nothing complicated or mysterious about this process. With your help and supervision, we are going to teach your children to use self-monitoring as a measure of their progress on the Stoplight Diet. It simply means teaching them to keep track of their own behavior — a valuable lesson that will give your children the skills to stay lean long after they have grown up and are off on their own.

Nowhere is self-monitoring more important than in keeping a record of body weight, exercise, and diet. Without self-monitoring, change is very difficult. How could anyone possibly know how much he or she has eaten without keeping track? Becoming aware of eating and exercise patterns is a necessary first step to changing habits. That is why you and your family will begin writing down what you eat each day, what you weigh, and how much you exercise.

Daily records of what your family eats will serve as a helpful reminder — a source of feedback, really — that tells you and your children how well you are doing on the Stoplight Diet. Daily weigh-ins, another means of self-monitoring, will show you an overall pattern of weight loss, even when the pounds do not drop off every day. And daily monitoring of exercise, which is discussed in Week 4, will help you increase physical activity and burn off excess calories.

In general, our studies of families on the Stoplight Diet show that self-monitoring has two main values:

· It helps make you and your family aware of what you eat and how much you exercise.
· It provides the motivation to continue working toward your goals. Watching the pounds drop off and seeing how your eating and exercise habits are changing provide a real sense of accomplishment.

Monitoring What You Eat

Foods consumed by your family will be recorded on a daily food chart and compiled in a habit book. This is a type of diary in which you log what and how much you eat, and when you consume it. Each person in your family will keep his or her own daily charts and collect them in an individual habit book. We recommend introducing the habit book as a fun project. Call it "The Stoplight Diary," and let your children design their own covers with crayons or colored pencils. Perhaps they would like to clip pictures from old magazines and make a collage cover. Whatever you do, make it fun and interesting for your children. Capture their imagination.

At the end of each day, you and your children will tally the totals and, like Monday-morning quarterbacks, see where you did well and where there is room for improvement. Appendix C is a blank form that can be used to record what you eat each day. At the University of Pittsburgh, a week's worth of such blank charts are distributed to every person participating in the Stoplight Diet program. We recommend that you do the same for your family. Have the form in appendix C photo-copied and enlarged to 8½ by 11 inches.

Figure 1 shows how a completed daily food chart might appear. Here's how to record what you eat:

· Fill in the name and date at the top of the page and the daily calorie-range goal in the box at the bottom.

· In the leftmost column, indicate when the food is eaten.

· Write down everything that you eat and drink, from your morning coffee (including, of course, the sugar and milk added) to your mid-night snack.

· Be sure to record the *amount* of food and beverages consumed. Portion sizes are very important. When they are inaccurate, they can be the source of "hidden calories." The best bet is to use measuring cups and spoons, but make sure that measurements are level — as in one *level* tablespoon, not one heaping tablespoon. We also recommend purchasing a couple of inexpensive measuring cups and spoons. Many families who tested the Stoplight Diet program at the University of Pittsburgh found that between food preparation and serving they needed the extra sets. Another recommendation: purchase a good kitchen scale. It need not be fancy or expensive, but it is vital for accurate measure-ment.

· In the spaces provided, indicate whether a food falls into the red, the yellow, or the green category. Refer to appendix B if necessary.

· Also keep track of how many servings from each of the Basic Four food groups you have eaten. A checkmark can be used to indicate one full serving. The Basic Four food category should be indicated for each food or left blank if a food doesn't fall into one of the Basic Four groups. As you record this information each day, your family will become more aware of proper nutrition.

· In the column labeled "Calories," write down the number per serving. "The Stoplight Diet Food Guide" (appendix B) contains a caloric listing of most foods. If you cannot find an item there, try looking on the food label. Many products now provide calorie counts; just be sure to check the serving size for an accurate calculation. You may also want to invest in one of the many handbooks for calorie-counters now on the market.

· Fill in the totals at the end of the day. Record the total number of red foods in the "Food Group Color" box.

Name _____ JAN _____   Date _WEDNESDAY, SEPT. 5_

Time	Food or Drink	Amount	Number of Calories	Food Group Color	Basic Four Food Group P	G	F&V	D
7:15 AM	SKIM MILK	1/4 C.	20	Y				1/4
	RICE KRISPIES	3/4 C.	80	Y		✓		
	STRAWBERRIES FRESH PLAIN	1/2 C.	26	Y			2/3	
	ORANGE JUICE FROZEN UNSWEETENED	1/2 C.	40	Y			✓	
	WHITE BREAD TOAST - PLAIN	1 SLICE	80	Y		✓		
12 NOON	AMERICAN CHEESE	1-OUNCE SLICE	100	Y				✓
	ITALIAN BREAD	2 SLICES	160	Y		2		
	MUSTARD	2 tsp	0	G				
	LETTUCE	1/2 C.	5	G			1/2	
	TOMATO (2-INCH DIAMETER)	1/2	10	G			1/2	
	WATERMELON FRESH UNSWEETENED	1/2 C.	20	Y			1/2	
	SKIM MILK	1/2 C.	40	Y				1/2
3:15 PM	WATER	1 C.	0	G				
5:30 PM	CHICKEN BREAST BROILED	3 oz.	150	Y	✓			
	CARROTS FROZEN BOILED	1/4 C.	10	G			1/2	
	SKIM MILK	1/2 C.	40	Y				1/2
	BROCCOLI FRESH PLAIN RAW	1/4 C.	10	G			1/2	
✱ AT GRANDMA'S	CHOCOLATE CAKE WITH WHITE ICING	1/2 SQUARE	180	R				
8:45 PM	HARD-BOILED LARGE EGGS	2	160	Y	✓			
Totals			1131	1R	2	4	4 7/6	2 1/4
Goals			900-1200		2	4	4	3

Figure 1   Sample Daily Food Chart

How to Record Food

Here are a few simple guidelines for recording accurately:

• Always write down what you eat or drink, and do so right after finishing a meal or a snack. Carry your habit book with you whenever possible, since foods that are not recorded are often forgotten. Encourage your children to do the same.

• Obviously, children who eat lunch at school may have to wait until they come home to log in what they ate during the day. One tip is to have them write down what they ate at school on a 3-by-5-inch card or on a piece of notebook paper. They can transfer the information to their habit books after school. Since they probably will not have access to a scale or measuring cups at school, they will have to estimate the portions they eat.

• If you pack a lunch for your child every day, you can jot down what you have prepared and compare it with what your child remembers eating. Better yet, have your son or daughter help you pack the lunch. Make sure whenever possible that your children measure food for themselves. There is no better way to learn about portion sizes.

• Record beverages in cups. Note whether the drink is a diet beverage, and in the case of milk, indicate the type — for instance, whole milk, 2-percent, or skim.

• The dairy group (indicated by *D* on the form) includes milk, hard cheese, yogurt, and ice cream or ice milk. (Ice cream and ice milk are red foods, however.) When recording cheeses, be specific. Write down the amount and type — for instance, 1 ounce American cheese, or ½ cup cottage cheese.

• Grains (indicated by a *G* on the form) include bread, cereal, pasta, pretzels, rice, rolls, crackers, and so forth.

• When recording bread, cookies, crackers, or rolls, be sure to write down the size, amount, and type of food.

• Cereals should be recorded in cups. Remember to note if sugar or fruit was added and be sure to write down the amount and kind of milk used.

• Eggs are considered protein and should be recorded under the column headed *P*. Note the number of eggs eaten, how they were cooked, and their size — for instance, small, medium, large, or jumbo. If you ate fried eggs, scrambled eggs, or an omelet, be sure to record any butter, margarine, or oil used in cooking, as well as any other ingredients, such as cheese, onions, milk, or meat.

• Meat should be weighed after cooking and recorded in ounces. If you want to err on the safe side, you can measure out 3 to 4 ounces of meat per family member, cook it, and then divide the meat portions equally among the number of people who will eat it. Meat, like eggs, counts as a protein serving.

• Certain foods served by the slice — pie, quiche, pizza, cake — are recorded by their dimensions. For example, one-eighth of a 9-inch pie or a 2-by-3-by-2-inch slice. Quiche and pizza are considered combination foods. How you log them on the food chart depends on their ingredients. For instance, a slice of cheese pizza would count as a grain (for the crust) and a dairy food (for the cheese).

• Cooked fruits and vegetables are usually measured by the cup: $\frac{1}{2}$ cup of broccoli; 1 cup of spinach. Large, raw fruit is recorded by size, such as 1 large apple. But smaller fruit, for example, berries or grapes, can be counted or measured by the cup. When in doubt, check "The Stoplight Diet Food Guide" (appendix B) for how to record a particular fruit or vegetable.

• Be sure to record anything added to the food during preparation or at the table. Butter on a potato is one example. Gravies, sauces, salad dressings, jellies, margarine, sugar, or sugar substitutes are others.

• If you or one of your children eats a red food, be sure to mark it with a star if it has been consumed outside the house. Remember: our studies show that people succeed much better on the Stoplight Diet if no red foods are kept in the house. Limit red foods to four or fewer per week — all eaten outside the home.

Make sure you and your children keep recording your food consumption. By remaining vigilant to what you are eating and when, you will discover your family's particular nutritional patterns and will be able to determine where changes need to be made. Keeping records will also remind you of what a terrific job you and your family are doing — providing what psychologists call *positive feedback*. With each day, you are learning the secrets of maintaining a well-balanced diet while decreasing what you eat in order to lose weight.

When the Williams family went on the Stoplight Diet, they turned food recording into a nightly ritual. "After dinner," Victoria Williams explains, "we would all linger at the table and pass around the guide as we wrote down what we ate for dinner. Sometimes we took turns looking up foods that we all ate. My husband would put on a big show. He would groan and say, 'How many calories is rice?' or 'Where do I look up the value for corn?' He'd make a big production about it.

"And the boys loved it," Victoria recalls. "They would giggle and show him how to look up the calorie counts for his food. Then we would add up our calories for the day and compare notes. It became something that we all looked forward to and enjoyed. And it gave us time together — really it was just five or ten minutes — but it gave us just a little extra time together before we all rushed off to regular weeknight activities."

Monitoring How Much You Weigh

Just as the daily food chart will give you and your family a measure of how many calories you are eating, the bathroom scale will show you how your new eating regimen is working on your waistlines.

It is important for everyone in the family to weigh in every day. The best time is either in the morning before breakfast or at night, just before bedtime. But no matter when you choose to weigh in, make sure that you do so consistently at the same time, since body weight generally fluctuates 1 to 2 pounds during the course of a day.

If you weigh yourself or your children in clothes, be sure that you wear the same clothes — or clothes of about the same weight — each time you step on the scale. The best way to keep track of your weight is by charting it every day. Figure 2 shows a filled-in daily weight chart, and appendix D provides a blank grid that can be photocopied for each member of the family.

Here is how to record weight:

• List the range of pounds in descending order from top to bottom along the left-hand vertical axis. Choose a range that allows you to record the present weight at a point about a quarter of the way from the top of the grid. You can use the grid to record weights to the nearest pound or half-pound.
• Record the date between the parentheses at the top of each column. (The chart is divided from left to right into vertical columns, one for each day of the week.)
• Record the weight each day in the box at the bottom of the column. Then place a dot or an X on the grid to indicate the daily weight.

Name ___SAM___ Week Number _1_

Goal Weight _101_

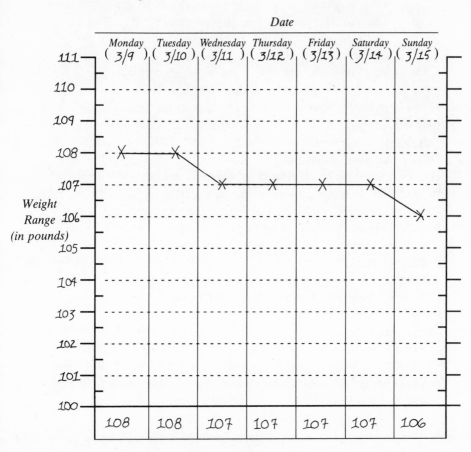

Figure 2   Sample Daily Weight Chart

• Connect the dots or X's as the week progresses to track any change in weight. (You may need to explain what a graph is to younger children, but this gives you a good opportunity to teach them an extra math lesson.)

Monitoring weight is one of the most important health habits on the Stoplight Diet, and it takes just one to two minutes a day. Families who charted their weight daily in the program conducted at the University of Pittsburgh were the most successful in achieving their goals.

Monitoring weight is also one of the most important means of maintaining weight loss once your children reach their ideal body weights. If you continue to encourage your children to chart their weight, both they and you will be aware of any increases and can quickly take action before unwanted pounds accumulate.

Now that you understand the Stoplight Diet signals and how to go about categorizing food, recording what you eat, and monitoring your weight, you can test your new knowledge with the following quiz. Also included are some practice exercises for calculating calories. You will find answers to the quiz at the end of the chapter. If you have any trouble answering a question, simply review the pertinent part of the chapter.

Once you are finished, pass the book to other family members. As you know, there is a companion chapter to this one written especially for your son or daughter. Like you, your children will test what they have learned with a quiz, which you can review with them. The more you and your children understand about the Stoplight Diet, the more successful you will be in achieving your weight-loss goals. Remember, you are joining 1,000 other family members who have already lost weight and built a healthier life-style through the Stoplight Diet.

Week 1 Quiz

1. The goal of most participants in the Stoplight Diet program is to _____ _____.

2. To lose weight, a person should _____ calorie intake and _____ physical activity.

3. The maximum amount of food that you are allowed to eat each day on the Stoplight Diet is your _____ _____.

4. The minimum number of calories that you should consume each day is _____. The minimum number of calories that a child the age of eight or older should consume is _____ calories.

5. Foods that are high in fat and sugar content are also high in _____.

6. What color category of foods should you avoid? _____

7. Which color of food is very low in calories and thus allows you to consume just about as much as you like? _____

8. Which color of food should be eaten in the most limited quantities each week? _____ How many servings per week of these foods can be consumed? _____ Where should they be eaten? _____

9. Foods that are deep-fried belong to the _____ color category.

10. Foods that are the mainstay of the Stoplight Diet are in the _____ color group. Foods in the _____ color category are relatively low in calories for the amount of nutrients they provide, but they are not quite as low in calories as green foods.

11. It is essential that you and your children eat a balanced diet made up of food from the _____ basic food groups.

12. The Basic Four food groups are _____, _____, _____, and _____.

13. A food that contains several different ingredients is called a _____ food. There are special rules for determining whether these foods are in the red or the yellow food category. One of the rules is that a dish falls in the red category if the combined calories in the ingredients add up to _____ or more per serving.

14. Combination foods that contain a red ingredient are categorized as a _____ food. Combination dishes that contain a yellow ingredient count as a _____ food if they include less than 350 calories.

To answer the following questions, use "The Stoplight Diet Food Guide" (appendix B). For each food listed, write the color category beside it.

Food	Color
15. Apple	_____
16. Two-percent milk	_____
17. Cottage cheese	_____
18. Carrots	_____
19. Soda crackers	_____
20. Baked chicken	_____
21. Fried chicken	_____
22. Doughnuts	_____
23. Peanut butter	_____
24. Diet margarine	_____

Answers

1. lose weight
2. decrease/increase
3. calorie limit
4. 900/900
5. calories
6. red
7. green
8. red/four/away from home

9. red
10. yellow/yellow
11. four
12. protein/grains/ fruits and vege- tables/dairy
13. combination/350
14. red/yellow
15. yellow

16. red
17. yellow
18. green
19. yellow
20. yellow
21. red
22. red
23. yellow
24. red

Week 2
The ABCs
of Nutrition

By now, you have cleaned the cupboards and tossed out all the red foods in your house. You have had a week to learn the Stoplight signals and, like most families on the Stoplight Diet, you and your children are beginning to watch the scale readings move downward, or at least stay at the same number of pounds.

At this time, you will start to feel the rhythm of the Stoplight Diet. Perhaps you notice that you now get on the scale each morning without thinking about it. Or maybe you catch yourself discussing red foods, yellow foods, and green foods with your children instead of talking about what you will have for dessert.

However it happens to you, this is the week that you and your family will start to feel and see some of the changes you are making.

If you are limiting calories, you may be surprised to find how much — and how well — you can eat on just 900 to 1,200 calories a day. You are probably learning to savor salads and to snack on fruit instead of candy. Many people find themselves packing lunch to take to the office and discover two benefits: they eat more healthfully and save money. At night, you may be among the Stoplight Diet families who dine on stir-fried foods — an excellent way to cut down on calories, saturated fats, and cholesterol while increasing your intake of vitamin-filled and fiber-rich vegetables. Or perhaps you have rediscovered the many varieties of pasta. This low-calorie, filling dish can change its flavor by a simple switch of sauces. Maybe your family is like those in our program who shaved calories by feasting on fish several nights a week instead of red meat or poultry. You can eat 3 ounces of shrimp or sole and consume just 100 calories — 120 calories less than an equivalent amount of beef, veal, pork, or lamb.

If you do not need to lose weight but are following the Stoplight Diet program to change eating habits and support your son's or daughter's quest to lose weight, you may be amazed at the wide variety of foods within the green and yellow categories. And rather than absentmindedly reaching for food, you may find yourself thinking about it first — a good indication that you are on the road to better nutrition.

This is also the week that you will begin to notice how familiar you are with the various food groups. By now, you have probably learned which color category each of your family's favorite meals fall into, and you know calorie counts for many foods without checking the food guide. Many families also report that by Week 2 they begin to measure portions of food automatically. What was a chore the week before starts to become rote — another marker that there is real behavior change under way.

You have probably noticed that your children are also getting into the groove.

"By the second week, our son Christopher was using a measuring cup to dole out his cornflakes and skim milk every morning without being asked," says Jeanne Smith, a trim, thirty-four-year-old professional who helped her ten-year-old stepson go from being a round-faced, roly-poly child to a lean young lad in six months. "Christopher was also very good about writing down what he ate."

Like the Smiths, however, you may have already discovered that parts of the program are harder than others for your children. "My husband and I struggled for a while to get Christopher on the scale every day," Jeanne recalls. "He really resisted doing that. He seemed to associate weighing himself with all the past disappointments of gaining weight, and I think he was afraid that he wouldn't be successful. But we just kept assuring him that if he stayed with the program, he would lose weight eventually, and we told him that the important thing was to get in the habit of weighing himself every day. It took some time, but now since he has seen the pounds drop off, he weighs himself every day without being reminded."

Each child on the Stoplight Diet will lose weight at his or her own pace. During the first week or two, your child is likely to achieve the most rapid weight loss — perhaps as much as 2 to 4 pounds. Such a quick initial decrease is typical of most weight-loss diets as the body adjusts to a new way of eating. But thereafter, the pounds may drop off more slowly. One week you may find that your child loses just half a pound. The next week, the scale may show a 1-pound loss. Some weeks, the scale may stay the same, only to drop by a pound or so the next week. Remember that the Stoplight Diet is designed for your child to lose weight slowly and safely. The goal is not just getting lean, but also changing eating and exercise habits forever. The American Heart Association advises: "Make [dietary] changes over a period of several months so they become a natural part of your permanent eating pattern." This is what you are helping your child to do on the Stoplight Diet.

If you run into some resistance to the program at your house, do not despair. Remember that it may take some time to change your children's habits. Remind your children that this diet is for them. Tell them again that the whole family is participating to help support them but that ultimately they have to want the change, and be willing to work for it.

Try not to be impatient. You should begin to see some change now, but as you know, each child is an individual and it takes some people longer to modify their behavior than others. You may find that you have to scale back your expectations of change in your child. Perhaps it will take your child an extra week to get into the rhythm of logging in what he or she eats every day.

If your daughter has trouble remembering to fill out her daily food record after each meal, remind her when you sit down to dinner that you will be filling out your own form right after the meal. Your daughter will learn from your example and is likely to join you as you complete your form. That's a much better lesson than nagging her to fill out her food form. If your son often forgets to weigh himself every day, remind him at breakfast what you weigh. Then ask if he has weighed himself yet. He will soon remember through your example to weigh himself every day.

In general, we have found that the majority of children succeed very well in our program as long as a parent also participates and supervises the child's progress. Problems do sometimes arise in families in which parents do not pay attention to the program or do not participate. It is very difficult for a child to have the motivation and interest to undertake the Stoplight Diet alone. The key to success is for the entire family to join in. We have also seen problems arise in families with caretakers. If you have a housekeeper, a regular baby-sitter, or a favorite relative who spends a significant portion of time with your children, make sure that that person understands and follows the Stoplight Diet program while overseeing your children. You may even want to ask your caretaker to read this book.

You and your children already know that to lose weight you have to eat fewer calories and exercise more. In fact, as mentioned earlier, to lose 1 pound, it is necessary to burn up 3,500 calories more than you eat. That means to lose 10 pounds, a person has to burn 35,000 calories more than he or she would normally.

When you decrease the number of calories eaten each day, it is important to eat wisely and guarantee proper nutrition. The Stoplight Diet is designed to promote weight loss while maintaining a well-balanced diet. But the program does not stop there. It is geared to reshape the eating habits of you and your family for a lifetime, not just for the weeks or months of weight loss.

It used to be that eating was a ritual — a way to stoke the inner furnace with energy needed during the day. Today, we know that food plays a far more important role than merely providing energy. And we now know more than ever the meaning of the nutrition adage "You are what you eat." Today, that saying is backed by evidence from numerous scientific studies that show the importance of diet in preventing serious illnesses such as cancer and heart disease.

High-fat diets — the traditional American diet ranks among the fattiest in the world — are associated with increased levels of cancer of the breast, colon, uterus, and prostate. And since high dietary fat puts on unwanted pounds and increases blood levels of cholesterol, these diets are also linked to an increased risk of heart attacks, stroke, and other cardiovascular diseases.

For these reasons, the National Cancer Institute, the American Heart Association, the National Academy of Sciences, and other respected medical organizations recommend important dietary changes to promote good health and lengthen life. By following the Stoplight Diet, you and your family are taking steps to follow these recommendations. We would like to emphasize during this second week some important guidelines that will lead you even farther down the road to good health.

First, by making these changes, your family is switching not to food martyrdom but back to the way Americans ate at the turn of the twentieth century. That means more potatoes (without butter or sour cream). Less red meat. More whole-grain foods, like oatmeal, pasta, and dark bread. Fewer whole-milk products, but more low-fat dairy foods. More fresh vegetables. More beans. More fresh fruit. Less junk food — particularly the 40 gallons of sugar-sweetened soda pop consumed by the average American in 1983. Junk foods boast few vitamins and minerals and are loaded with sugar and fat — both sources of concentrated calories.

Just making these changes automatically helps cut calories. But couple this turn-of-the-century style of eating with the calorie limits of the Stoplight Diet and your son or daughter will be headed toward a leaner way of life.

Our studies show that the children who follow the nutritional recommendations and change their eating habits lose weight and maintain their new, trim figures more easily. For instance, we found that children who eat the least amount of red foods do best at losing weight. And upon examining why these children ate fewer red foods than their peers, we discovered a reason: they had received more parental support for losing weight in our program.

Explain to your children that good nutrition means eating a well-balanced diet — one that supplies the important nutrients their bodies need for good health, energy, and growth. Children of all ages can benefit from this lesson. We have found it particularly helpful to explain to young children that their bodies are like a furnace. Food is the fuel that keeps the body running. Calories help us measure how much fuel we are using. Exercise is a way to turn up the body's furnace.

We also explain that losing weight is a matter of nutritional balance. Simple as it seems, dieters often forget this principle — and that is one reason why so many of them fail. They cut back on calories to an extreme and eat an unbalanced diet, often lacking in adequate amounts of carbohydrates, fiber, vitamins, and minerals. Since their diet has taught them a lot about sacrifice but little about nutrition and even less about changing behavior, these dieters quickly revert to their old eating habits once they have lost the pounds they wanted to shed. Since they have no new behavior to rely upon, the pounds get put right back on. We do not want you or your children to experience this yo-yo effect. The Stoplight Diet has been carefully designed to help avoid this situation.

One way to prevent the yo-yo effect is to ensure that your children's diet represents a proper mix from what we call the Basic Four food groups — protein, grains, fruits and vegetables, and dairy. This is the plan that you learned about in the first week of the Stoplight Diet. In this, the second week, we are going to help you increase your nutritional knowledge, and that of your children, about the Basic Four food groups.

If you guide your family in their choice of foods from these four food groups, you will be teaching them how to eat in a balanced, nutritious way. If you also show them the importance of eating the recommended number of servings from each food group, you will ensure that they get the nutrients they need — even while losing weight. The table below will help you guide your family to a balanced diet.

One crucial rule to stress to your children: Never skimp on the allotted number of daily calories. Everyone eight years old or older must eat at least 900 calories a day, and six- and seven-year-olds should have no less than 1,000 calories daily. Eating below those minimums makes it difficult to take in the number of recommended servings essential for proper nutrition, good health, and necessary growth. But with some careful choices — and your guidance — your children can eat very healthfully.

Once your children have eaten the minimum daily number of calories, they may choose to eat the remaining calories, up to a total of 1,200 a day, from among whatever green or yellow foods best fit their eating preferences and meet with your approval. And it is all right if they do not want the additional 200 or 300 calories some days.

Once again, the key points are to make sure that your children do not eat less than 900 or 1,000 calories every day (depending on their age) and that they eat the recommended number of servings of food from each of the Basic Four food groups.

BASIC FOUR FOOD GROUP MINIMUM CALORIE GUIDELINES

Food Group	Recommended Number of Servings per Day	Size of Serving	Calorie Range per Serving	Calorie Range per Day
Protein (P)	2	2 ounces	67–147	134–294
Grains (G)	4	1 slice of bread, ½–¾ cup of cereal, or ½ cup of cooked rice or pasta	80	320
Fruits and vegetables (F&V)	4	1 small piece of fruit, ½–⅔ cup of vegetables, or ½ cup of juice	20–40	80–160
Dairy (D)	3	1 cup	80	240

Protein (P)

There is a widespread misconception in the United States about protein. Most people think that high-protein foods are nonfattening. At the same time, they consider high-carbohydrate foods — for instance, bread, potatoes, pasta, rice, and beans — as the major culprits behind added body weight. How many times have you heard people say, "No bread for me, thanks, I'm trying to take off a few pounds"? Meanwhile, they heap their plates full of steak because "it's high in protein and good for me."

Nothing could be further from the truth. The person who tries to save calories by passing up a baked potato or a piece of bread or a helping of rice for a huge portion of red-meat "protein" makes a poor choice. A 9-ounce T-bone steak contains about 660 calories, while a slice of bread or a small baked potato has just 80 calories. In the steak, about 20 percent of those calories come from protein, but a large percentage of the remaining calories are fat — mostly saturated fat that helps raise blood levels of cholesterol. If you teach your children this important lesson about protein, you will go a long way in helping them avoid unnecessary calories.

You also need to teach them that a gram of protein or of carbohydrate contains just 4 calories, while a gram of fat contains 9 calories — more than twice as much.

Beef is not the only meat to contain fat. Lamb, pork, and veal contain roughly the same percentage of fat as beef. Even poultry contains a significant portion of fat. For instance, consume 4 ounces of roasted chicken breast, including the skin, and you will have eaten about 36 of every 100 calories, or 36 percent, as fat. But eat the same amount of roasted chicken breast *without* the skin and only 19 percent — 19 of every 100 calories — comes from fat.

Consumption of large amounts of red meat and poultry is one major reason why the average American diet is known worldwide for being extra high in fat and protein. Most Americans eat about double the amount of protein that they need. Too much protein can strain the kidneys. High-protein diets also "may be associated with an increased risk of cancer at certain sites" in the body, according to a 1982 report published by the National Academy of Sciences. Among the cancers linked to high-protein diets (and note that the key word is "linked," not "proved") are cancers of the breast, intestine, and pancreas.

Since animal proteins — eggs, cheese, milk products, red meat, and poultry — also contain large amounts of fat, some scientists believe that this could account for the higher incidence of cancer associated with high-protein diets.

Exceptions to this close relationship between fat and protein are proteins derived from plants and vegetables rather than from animals. Beans, lentils, and other legumes are high in protein yet low in fat and relatively low in calories. Like animal-derived protein, these plant-source proteins can provide niacin and thiamine, two important nutrients. What they lack, however, is iron — the mineral necessary for strong red blood cells. The message, then, is not to give up red meat, but to consume it in moderation. *New York Times* health and nutrition columnist Jane Brody says that a new, more healthful way of thinking about red meat and poultry is to view them as another type of condiment. You can do this by serving meat in just 2- or 3-ounce portions, mixed with pasta, beans, or rice, or in numerous other combinations. Contrary to popular belief, these portions will be large enough to supply sufficient protein and other essential nutrients, but small enough to limit calories and saturated fat.

Another good protein source is fish. Low in fat and calories, fish and seafood are wonderful alternatives to red meat, poultry, and other animal-derived proteins such as dairy products (which, as mentioned, usually contain lots of saturated fat and cholesterol).

In the last several years, scientists have discovered another health benefit of fish: fish oil. We now know that the oil of fish, particularly saltwater fish, contains a healthful class of substances called omega-3 fatty acids. It is these fatty acids that help explain how Alaskan Eskimos and Dutch fishermen can eat high-fat diets yet show little evidence of the heart disease and strokes that afflict other populations. These substances also seem to account for the lower incidence of breast cancer among Japanese women who live near the seacoast and eat a lot of fish as compared with their countrywomen who live inland.

Recent research suggests that eating two or three servings a week of oily ocean fish — salmon, mackerel, sable, crab, shrimp, tuna, and lobster, among others — has many health-promoting effects, including lowered risk of heart disease and inflammatory diseases such as arthritis. Omega-3 fatty acids also are effective in lowering certain kinds of blood cholesterol — especially one of the most dangerous types, known as LDL (low-density lipoprotein). So, when possible, incorporate fish into the Stoplight Diet, as a way of saving calories, adding variety, and promoting good health.

By adhering to these guidelines for consuming protein, your family will be following the recommendation to cut dietary fat proposed by the National Institutes of Health and the American Heart Association. The goal of these organizations is for Americans to reduce the percentage of fat in their diets to 30 percent or less of total calories. That is about a 10-percent reduction from the standard American diet.

Grains (G)

When you and your family begin cutting back on protein and fat, you will naturally reach for other foods to take their place. One of the best groups of foods to choose is the grain group.

Contrary to popular opinion, foods in the grain group are generally not fattening — unless, of course, you slather them with butter, margarine, cream cheese, or some other high-calorie spread. Exceptions to the generally low-calorie grain foods include bread and cereal products with a high fat or sugar content. Among these are granola, doughnuts, cakes, sweet rolls, and sugar-coated cereals that fall into the category of red foods.

What most foods in the grain group do provide, however, is iron (important for the oxygen-carrying red blood cells), B vitamins (needed for normal functioning of the nervous system), and protein (key to growth and good health). Moreover, many products in the grain food group are labeled "enriched," which means that the iron and B vitamins lost in certain kinds of food processing have been replaced.

Depending on what choices you make in the grain group, these foods can also add significant amounts of fiber to your family's diet — an important health recommendation from the National Cancer Institute. The average American consumes about 10 to 20 grams a day of fiber. Yet studies of populations throughout the world show that people who eat twice this amount of fiber have a lower rate of cancers of the colon and rectum. Based on these findings, the National Cancer Institute recommends that your family's diet provide at least 25 to 35 grams of fiber a day.

How much fiber you aim for depends on body size. Children may eat the recommended amount of fiber at the lower end of the range, while larger individuals need to aim for the upper end. To meet these new requirements, you must eat several servings a day of fiber-rich foods: breads and cereals made from whole grains, plus fruits and vegetables.

Fiber is nondigestible or partially digestible material produced by plant cells. Different types of fiber seem to vary in the health protection they offer. For instance, studies suggest that wheat bran, the kind found in most high-fiber products today, offers protection against colon cancer and some other intestinal disorders. Oat bran fiber, on the other hand, seems to have more global physiological effects, including lowering blood cholesterol levels, enhancing the body's absorption of sugar, and, in some cases, lowering blood pressure. In a study conducted at the Massachusetts Institute of Technology, researchers found that when students incorporated 1½ ounces of oat bran fiber into their diets, their blood cholesterol levels dropped 9 percent, even though they were eating more high-fat and high-cholesterol foods than usual. By comparison, wheat bran did not affect blood levels of cholesterol.

What does it mean to have a 9 percent reduction in blood cholesterol? For middle-aged men, it translates to an 18 percent reduction in the risk of heart attack, experts say. For people in their twenties, the benefits are even greater, perhaps rising to a 30-percent decrease in the risk of early heart attack, authorities estimate. The American Heart Association (which advocates consuming no more than 300 milligrams of cholesterol a day) notes that the 1968 National Heart Study showed that a low-fat, reduced-cholesterol diet "would reduce [blood] cholesterol in a large group of free-living adults. A similar diet consumed by children should produce comparable effects."

How do you add more fiber to your family's diet? Choose whole-grain products in place of refined white-flour foods. You can do this by encouraging your children to eat whole-wheat crackers; whole-wheat English muffins and bagels; and rye, whole-wheat, oatmeal, or pumpernickel bread.

A nutritious way to start the day is with high-fiber cereals at breakfast. But remember to avoid those that contain large amounts of high-calorie dried fruits, such as raisins. When in doubt, check the label. High-fiber cereals now tout their added fiber (a smart marketing tool). Your child can eat two-thirds of a cup of shredded wheat with extra bran and consume 10 grams of fiber, almost half the amount he or she needs to eat for the day. Add some fresh fruit on top and the fiber tally will increase another 1 or 2 grams. High-fiber cereals are sometimes not as appealing to children as low-fiber varieties. One option is to mix high-fiber cereals with low-fiber ones, keeping a close eye on total number of calories.

Other foods that can help your family increase their fiber intake include corn, popcorn (unbuttered, of course), tortillas, and whole-grain pasta. Dried beans are also a good source of fiber. Remember, it is best to consume at least four servings of grain a day.

Fruits and Vegetables (F&V)

Fruits and vegetables are generally low in calories yet have the added benefit of being loaded with vitamins, minerals, and fiber; they make a smart nutritional addition to any weight-loss diet. A well-balanced diet includes a minimum of four servings a day from the fruit-and-vegetable group.

(Some children strongly dislike vegetables. One way to overcome that problem is to make a game out of eating a new vegetable every day. We recommend keeping a "star chart" for younger children. Each time they eat a new vegetable, reward them with a gummed star or similar sticker on the chart. Another tactic is to require children to eat just three bites of a new vegetable. We do not believe in the "Clean Plate Club" approach. Children should not be forced to eat everything on their plates. They should eat until they are full. We are aware that many children will suddenly feel very full when the only food left on their plates is a helping of cooked carrots. Yet, given the opportunity, these same children will gladly eat another portion of meat or potatoes. We recommend that you require your children to try new foods — especially vegetables. We have found the three-bite rule to be quite effective in getting children who otherwise scorn vegetables to eat a small portion of them. Of course, these same children should never be allowed to have extra servings of other foods if they have not finished their vegetables.)

The only way to get into high-calorie trouble with fruits and vegetables is to deep-fry them in fat, slather them with butter, margarine, or some other high-calorie topping, or serve them with fattening sauces or syrups. To see how such additions can quickly add up, consider these examples:

• One-half cup of steamed carrots contains only 20 calories, while one-half cup of candied carrots has 60 calories — three times higher.

•   One-half cup of mashed potatoes runs 80 calories, versus 140 calories for one-half cup of french fries.

•   One-third cup of canned pineapple in its juice has 40 calories, while one-half cup of pineapple in heavy syrup runs 100 calories.

•   One-half cup of steamed green beans contains 20 calories; but serve the same amount of beans with 1 teaspoon of margarine and the calories triple.

Aside from being good, low-fat food choices, fruits and vegetables are also the largest suppliers of vitamins A and C. To repeat, it is important to eat at least four servings a day from this key food group. That can mean drinking 4 ounces of orange juice at breakfast, having a salad and half cup of strawberries at lunch, and eating broccoli at dinner.

Which fruits and vegetables you choose to buy and cook for your family can also make a big difference in health risk. The National Cancer Institute and the National Academy of Sciences report that diets high in vitamin C reduce the risk of developing cancers of the stomach and esophagus, while diets high in vitamin A cut the chances of developing cancer of the lung, bladder, and larynx.

Based on this evidence, the National Cancer Institute recommends that you and your family choose foods daily from the following list of produce that is high in these important vitamins. You will note that all of these foods are consistent with the Stoplight Diet, so you can help your children trim calories *and* eat more healthfully. The general rule is that sources of vitamin A are easy to recognize because they are generally fruits or vegetables that are yellow or orange or green in color. (An exception to this rule are oranges, which as a citrus fruit contain vitamin C but no vitamin A.)

Among the many sources of vitamins A and C are these foods:

•   Dark-green leafy vegetables such as broccoli, swiss chard, kale, spinach, romaine, endive, chicory, watercress, and collard, beet, mustard, and dandelion greens.

•   Green, yellow, and red peppers, asparagus, cauliflower, cabbage, brussels sprouts, bean sprouts, mushrooms, green beans, onions, okra, and tomatoes.

•   Yellow-orange vegetables such as carrots, sweet potatoes, pumpkin, and winter squash.

• Yellow-orange and other fleshy fruits, including apricots, berries, cantaloupes and other melons, cherries, papayas, peaches, plums, prunes, and pineapples.
• Citrus fruits such as lemons, limes, oranges, tangerines, tangelos, and grapefruit, or their natural juices.

In addition to rich amounts of vitamins and fiber, one family of vegetables also contains high levels of two substances that have been found to prevent the formation of intestinal tumors in laboratory animals. These substances, called indoles and isothiocyanates, are found in brussels sprouts, cabbage, broccoli, cauliflower, and rutabagas and other turnips — all members of the *cruciferous* vegetable family. Cruciferous vegetables are part of the mustard family. They grow wild in Europe and Asia and are noted for their strong odors, arising from sulfur compounds. The varieties of cruciferous vegetables that we know and eat are mutants of their wild ancestors.

The National Cancer Institute (NCI) and the National Academy of Sciences (NAS) recommend that you and your family consume cruciferous vegetables at least three times a week. NCI scientists are currently engaged in studies to identify and extract the protective chemicals from cruciferous vegetables.

Dairy (D)

The dairy food group contains a wide range of great-tasting foods and beverages, from cheese to whole milk to yogurt. These foods are excellent sources of calcium, phosphorus, and vitamin D. But they can also be high in calories, largely because they are high in saturated fat. Whole-milk products are also loaded with cholesterol, which means that these foods can help contribute to the development of heart disease and other cardiovascular problems.

Fortunately, there is a solution to this nutritional dilemma: skim milk. Skim milk comes close to being a nutritionally perfect food. It is rich in protein, low in fat, and high in calcium, phosphorus, and vitamin D — the minerals and vitamins necessary for strong bones.

Your children need to consume at least 24 ounces a day of skim milk to meet their calcium requirement, which is 900 milligrams of calcium per day. (Each 8-ounce glass of skim milk contains about 300 milligrams of calcium.) During this time in their lives, their skeletal systems are developing and they require sufficient amounts of calcium to form strong bones. Adults too need calcium. In particular, women begin losing calcium from their bones at about age thirty-five, a natural physiological process that accelerates after menopause and frequently leads to the degenerative bone disease known as osteoporosis.

Drinking skim milk — or consuming skim milk products — is an excellent way to obtain enough calcium each day. The 300 milligrams of calcium in each 8-ounce glass of skim milk (or buttermilk) is the highest amount of calcium available from any milk source. By comparison, whole milk and its many food by-products contain much less calcium. For instance, your son or daughter would have to eat 14 ounces of ice cream — 1¾ cups, at a whopping 455 calories — to get the same amount of calcium contained in just one 8-ounce glass of skim milk. And at just 80 calories, the skim milk is also an important calorie-saver. The accompanying table shows how much your children would have to eat of various milk products to match the amount of calcium in the one glass of skim milk.

Despite the many advantages of skim milk, it is also important not to allow children to drink unlimited quantities. Children who drink too much skim milk usually do so at the expense of other very nutritious foods, and the point of the Stoplight Diet is to learn how to eat well-balanced meals rather than overconsume any one food, even if it is good for you. That is why we recommend three 8-ounce servings a day from the dairy food group.

Cheese is another popular choice from the dairy group, but it must be eaten with caution. Cheese is far higher in calories and fat than skim

MILK AND DAIRY FAT PRODUCTS CONTAINING 300MG OF CALCIUM

	Amount	Number of Calories	Food Group Color
Skim milk	8 oz./1 cup	80	yellow
Buttermilk	8 oz./1 cup	80	yellow
Plain yogurt (low-fat)	8 oz./1 cup	140	yellow
American cheese	1½ oz./⅕ cup	150	yellow
Cheddar cheese	1½ oz./⅕ cup	150	yellow
Creamed cottage cheese	16 oz./2 cups	400	yellow
Half-and-half	8 oz./1 cup	320	red
Ice cream	14 oz./1¾ cups	455	red
Chocolate milk	8 oz./1 cup	250	red

milk or other skim milk products. On average, cheese contains about 100 calories per ounce, of which at least 50 percent (and usually far more) comes from pure fat. You can have your cheese and eat it too, however, by switching to low-fat cheeses that are made in part from skim milk. Many companies now make good-tasting skim-milk cottage cheese that contains about the same number of calories and amount of fat as skim milk.

Fat and high sugar content are the reasons why other well-liked dairy foods count as red foods. Among these are ice cream, pudding, and sweetened, whole-milk yogurt. Not only are these foods loaded with fat and sugar, but they also contain small amounts of calcium in proportion to their high calorie counts — three important factors that make them inappropriate choices for people who are trying to lose weight. (Plain yogurt made from skim milk is sold in supermarkets or can be made at home. Eaten alone, used in sauces and salad dressings, or mixed with fruit, plain yogurt is a good alternative to skim milk.)

Finally, cream, cream cheese, butter, sour cream, and margarine are often thought of as milk products. But since these foods contain little or no calcium and are really fats, they are excluded from the dairy group on the Stoplight Diet. If they are eaten, they must be recorded as a red food, and, of course, should not be kept in the home. When cooking, use just 1 to 2 teaspoons of vegetable oil. (A daily serving of fat can be 1 to 2 teaspoons of vegetable oil or 1 tablespoon of salad dressing.)

For quick reference, the Basic Four food groups are listed in appendix E along with the primary nutrients they provide. You will also find there the major food sources in each group and the number and size of daily servings recommended for a nutritious diet. Remember, to meet the nutritional needs for good health, adequate energy, and proper growth, it is important to eat according to the basic diet each day. To help you pick foods from the Basic Four food groups while staying within the calorie limits on the Stoplight Diet, we have assembled several sample menus in appendix F.

Vitamin Supplements

The Stoplight Diet is designed to provide enough nourishment from a variety of foods so that almost all vitamin and mineral supplements are unnecessary. If you and your family follow the Basic Four food guidelines each day, you probably will not need any supplements. The one exception is iron. Studies show that many women and children in the United States fall short of getting the recommended daily allowance of iron, an important mineral necessary for good blood formation. For this reason, you may want to consider giving your children iron supplements. Before taking any vitamins or minerals — and before giving them to your children — consult with your family physician or pediatrician. Taking too many vitamins, especially the fat-soluble vitamins A, D, E, and K, can be harmful to your health. Unlike water-soluble vitamins — the

---

TIPS ON NUTRITION

· Decrease fat in the diet wherever possible. Hidden fat crops up in many meat and milk products (unless they are made from skim milk). Trim all fat from meat before cooking. Eat all poultry without the skin, and try to consume more white meat — which is lower in fat — than dark meat. Eat fish and legumes more often.

· Choose more "complex carbohydrates" for grain products. These whole-grain foods are good sources of fiber. When counting calories, remember that foods in the grains group are usually equivalent to — not higher than — foods in the protein group.

· Choose fresh fruits and vegetables over canned products, which can be higher in calories. In most cases, fresh produce also contains greater amounts of vitamins and minerals, since nutrients can be lost in canning or other food processing.

· Avoid eating too much food from the protein group. Once you have eaten the minimum of two 2-ounce servings a day, foods consumed from this group will be stored as fat.

· Make sure that enough grains are consumed, but omit the high-calorie extras, like dried fruit in cereals or rich sauces on pasta.

· Remember that skim milk (or buttermilk) contains more calcium per serving than any other food or beverage.

· Eat plenty of fruits and vegetables, which are higher in nutrients yet lower in calories than foods in the other three basic food groups.

B vitamins and vitamin C — which are flushed from your system, fat-soluble vitamins are stored in fat cells throughout the body. That means that they can quickly rise to toxic levels and cause damage to the body.

A Word about Snacks and Fast Food

Excellent snacks on the Stoplight Diet include carrot and celery sticks (which are low in calories yet high in fiber), slices of raw zucchini or cucumber, and rice cakes (just 35 calories per cake). Popcorn made with a little vegetable oil and served unbuttered, with little or no salt, is just 40 calories per cup and is another good snack. It also contains a moderate amount of fiber. Air-popped corn is even lower in calories. Pretzels are another acceptable snack, provided that they are eaten in limited quantities.

Looking for a special hot-weather treat? Try making your own frozen fruit bars by freezing juice in ice cube trays. Frozen, unsweetened fruit mixed with skim milk yogurt is another refreshing summer snack or dessert. To stretch cool drinks, mix 1 or 2 ounces of fruit juice with about 6 ounces of carbonated water. You can serve four to eight of these drinks to your children for the calorie cost of one 8-ounce glass of juice.

In today's busy world, almost every family eats some meals outside the home, often in fast-food restaurants. Although we do not advocate relying on these restaurants for good nutrition, we recognize that many families on the Stoplight program find themselves eating several times a month in fast-food establishments. It is possible to eat wisely when you and your family are faced with dining on fast food. That is why we include a fast-food section in the Stoplight Diet Food Guide (appendix B). Use this section to help your family make good choices when they eat out.

Week 2 Quiz

1. Well-balanced diets are important for everyone, but they are especially important for children because children are _____.

2. On the Stoplight Diet, you and your family learn how to lose weight and how to _____ your eating habits.

3. To guarantee that you and your family consume balanced and nutritionally sound meals, it is important to eat a number of servings

from each of the Basic Four food groups. Circle the minimum number of daily servings from each group.

a. Dairy   1 2 3 4 5
b. Protein   1 2 3 4 5
c. Fruits and vegetables 1 2 3 4 5
d. Grains   1 2 3 4 5

Answer true or false:

4. People who consume diets high in animal protein simultaneously consume high amounts of fat.

5. As a rule, bread, pasta, crackers, rice, and other foods in the grains group are not higher in calories than foods in the protein group.

6. Skim milk is a good source of calcium yet is low in fat.

7. Eating a balanced diet is difficult if you consume less than _____ calories each day.

8. Healthy children who eat a balanced diet usually do not need a _____ supplement.

In the following list, indicate whether each food is considered as protein (P), grains (G), fruits and vegetables (F&V), or dairy (D). Then show which color it counts as on the Stoplight Diet — red, yellow, or green.

Food	Basic Four Food Group	Color
9. Rye bread		
10. Poached egg		
11. American cheese		
12. Peas		
13. Whole milk		
14. Turkey		
15. Salmon (uncanned)		
16. Shrimp		
17. Avocado		
18. Raisins		
19. Croissant		
20. Corned beef		
21. Bagel		

Answers

1. growing
2. change
3. a. 3
   b. 2
   c. 4
   d. 4
4. True
5. True

6. True
7. 900
8. vitamin
9. G/yellow
10. P/yellow
11. D/yellow
12. F&V/yellow
13. D/red

14. P/yellow
15. P/yellow
16. P/yellow
17. F&V/red
18. F&V/red
19. G/red
20. P/red
21. G/yellow

Week 3
Praise and
Rewards

Everyone loves praise. Employees enjoy hearing from their bosses when they do a great job. Students like the praise of teachers. And children adore receiving praise from their parents. It gives them recognition, satisfaction, reassurance, and, most of all, tells them that their parents are pleased with their behavior.

Praise works wonders for encouraging a multitude of good behaviors in children: Studying. Doing chores. Making beds. Keeping their rooms clean. Being home on time. And one of the most effective uses of praise is in shaping good eating and exercise habits.

For this reason, praise is an integral part of the Stoplight Diet. You and your spouse will encourage and support your sons or daughters in many ways as they lose weight, but one of the most important is by praising them for their good behavior on this program. Our studies of the Stoplight Diet demonstrate time and time again that frequent praise by parents helps children stick with the program and lose weight for good. When we compared two identical groups of children but instructed the parents of only one group to give praise to their children, the results were surprisingly different. Five months after starting the diet, the children who received praise from their parents for adhering to the program lost three times the amount of weight lost by the children who were not rewarded with praise. Quite simply, praise works.

What is so special about praise? How is it that a few words here and there, a hug, a high-five, or a pat on the back can evoke such wonders? Simple. Praise is a motivator. Everyone feels better after being praised. Think about it: Which would you rather hear? Words of praise or negative criticism? Few, if any, adults would choose the latter. The same holds true for children.

Human nature also dictates that once you have been praised you like to be praised again. To earn that praise, you will repeat whatever behavior prompted it. Psychologists call this process *positive reinforcement.* Thus, the child who is told what a great job he or she has done in filling out the Stoplight Diet habit chart will be likely to fill it out again. And if you mention how pleased you are that your son or daughter limited red foods to four or fewer this week, he or she will be inclined to do so next week. Telling your child how proud you are of a specific behavior encourages its continuation.

Praise also helps children feel good about themselves — and a strong self-image is important. Praise is especially beneficial for overweight children, who often suffer from low self-esteem. In using praise, you rely on what psychologists consider one of the best management techniques a parent can use.

Nightly Family Meetings

On the Stoplight Diet, one of the ways to guarantee that your children get the praise they need is to schedule a nightly family meeting. Each evening, either you or your spouse — or both of you — should sit down with your children, review their daily charts, and praise their progress.

This meeting need not take long. Most parents budget just five or ten minutes, but it is essential that you meet briefly every night with your children. Many families in our program met after dinner and made a ritual of filling out the Stoplight Diet charts together and then reviewing them.

Some families decide that just one parent will talk with the children. Others set aside a few minutes to talk before their children go to bed. However you choose to do it, our key message is that you must meet every day. Make sure that you meet in a comfortable place, free from the distractions of television, stereos, and phones. Give a few minutes of undivided attention to your children.

Be positive during these meetings. Be sure to praise each child's *behavior.* It is not enough to tell your child after the nightly-meeting review, "I'm proud of you." Be specific and tell your son that you are proud of the way he recorded his food every day or compliment your daughter's request for a green food instead of a red food at snack time.

It is also very easy to unwittingly mix praise and criticism. The result is a confusing message for your child, like the one given by the mother in the following conversation.

MOTHER: Let's see how you did today, Elizabeth. I see that you recorded your food as you should. That's very good. It makes me very pleased that you are logging in what you eat. You also ate less than 1,200 calories. That's very good, honey.

ELIZABETH: Thanks, Mom.

MOTHER: But I also see that you did not weigh yourself today. How can you expect to keep track of your weight if you don't get on the scale every day? If you are this careless, it can carry over to everything that you do. You are going to have to do better than this, young lady!

In this case, the mother did a very good job of praising her daughter's behavior at the beginning of the meeting, but she undid all her good efforts with her final comments. Elizabeth received a message filled with criticism that says her mother does not accept her behavior. This kind of a message does not help to build Elizabeth's self-image, and it is really undeserved, given the good work that Elizabeth did on this particular day. The mother forgot to offer constructive criticism, to provide encouragement for Elizabeth to be more diligent about recording her weight. Here is how she could have responded to Elizabeth in a more positive way:

MOTHER: Let's see how you did today, Elizabeth. I see that you recorded your food as you should. That's very good. It makes me very pleased that you are logging in what you eat. You also ate less than 1,200 calories. That's also very good, honey. You are doing an excellent job sticking with the Stoplight Diet. I am very proud.

ELIZABETH: Thanks, Mom.

MOTHER: But there's one thing missing here. I don't see your weight recorded for today. Did you do that?

ELIZABETH (*looking downcast*): No, I forgot to weigh myself today.

MOTHER: I'm disappointed, but I am sure you know how important it is to keep track of your weight. You are doing such a good job with what you eat. I think if you get on the scale every day you will be pleased to see how your weight is changing. Let's make a pact to weigh ourselves together for the next couple of mornings until you get back into the swing of things. How about meeting me in the bathroom tomorrow morning at seven o'clock?

ELIZABETH (*brightening*): Okay, Mom. I'd like that.

MOTHER (*as she gives Elizabeth a hug*): I'm really proud of the way you wrote down your food and stayed within the calorie range, Elizabeth. You are doing a very good job.

In this second conversation, you can see that Elizabeth's mother expressed her disappointment, but she avoided nagging or yelling at her daughter. Yelling and nagging sometimes decrease bad behavior but they do not increase good behavior, which is one of the goals of our program.

You can see that this mother also made sure that she gave Elizabeth praise for the good work she did on the Stoplight Diet. At the same time, she showed Elizabeth how she could do better, and offered to help her do so.

If you take this approach with your children, you too can successfully motivate them to stay with the Stoplight Diet. Remember, it takes time to change behavior, but before you know it, you will see results. We recommend that you praise your children for behavior changes — not just for losing weight. Every dieter reaches a plateau and may not lose weight one week. By praising your children's behavior — rather than the weight loss — you reinforce their new eating and exercise and self-monitoring habits. Instead of saying to your daughter, "Gee, I'm glad that you lost a pound this week," you can say, "Gee, I'm glad that you watched what you ate and exercised this week so that you could lose a pound. That must make you feel very good."

The nightly meeting also allows you to keep track of how your children are faring on the Stoplight Diet. You will be able to gauge their understanding of the various red, yellow, and green food groupings. Are they keeping within the allotted calorie ranges, and are they eating balanced diets? You may want to spot-check a few calorie counts to make sure that your children have recorded the values accurately.

Do your children drink enough milk and consume enough grains, fruits and vegetables, and protein daily? Double-check what they have listed under the Basic Four food groups to be sure. You should also make sure that your children understand the concept of portions. Do they measure their food? Are they recording all that they eat? For instance, did they forget to write down the mayonnaise on their sandwich at school or the bun they ate with their burger? These are both easy to miss.

One mother discovered at the nightly meetings that her son was having difficulty learning the red, yellow, and green foods. To help teach him, she took "The Stoplight Diet Food Guide" along with her when she went to the grocery store. Every time her son requested a food, she had him look it up in the guide. It helped him learn to categorize his favorite foods and it made him more aware of calorie counts. Soda pop (95 calories per cup) was replaced by orange juice (80 calories per cup), a lower-calorie but still well-liked substitute. Her son made the choices, learned why they were the right ones, and did not complain about what she brought home from the store. Grocery shopping switched from being a struggle to a pleasant outing for the two of them.

There are other fringe benefits of the nightly meeting. One mother found that it allowed her to check on her son's spelling and handwriting progress — both needed some improvement. One father used the nightly meeting as an opportunity for a math lesson. Tallying the foods eaten and the calories consumed each day gave his daughter extra practice in addition.

The nightly meeting also gives you a chance to share your own progress with your children. After you have looked over your son's or daughter's daily food record, offer yours for checking. Your child will see that the two of you share the same goals. If you do not need to lose weight, you can emphasize how you are changing your eating habits. Show how you are staying within the calorie-intake range that is appropriate for you and that you are limiting yourself to four or fewer red foods each week — always eaten away from home. It is important for children trying to lose weight on the Stoplight Diet to know that they have a partner — and a role model — in you and the rest of your family. They will quickly learn that the family is participating in the program together.

Rules for Giving Praise

As mentioned, a key benefit of the nightly meeting is the opportunity to offer encouragement and praise to your son or daughter. By positively reinforcing their behavior, you will help shape their new habits. Remember that praise means more than being nice. To work as the best possible motivator for your children, praise should be offered according to the suggestions given below. Parents who participated in our program found that these "rules" were particularly helpful.

• *Rule 1: Describe the behavior you are praising specifically; keep your comments brief.*
The nightly meetings usually should take no more than five to ten

minutes a night. We are sure that you have many other activities that you need to do every evening, and your child is likely to lose interest if the meetings drag on much more than a few minutes. Think of these meetings as you would a meeting with your boss. Keep them brief and to the point.

You can lavish praise by using just a few carefully chosen words. Try to describe what your child did and why you appreciate it. Being specific is important. It means that your child will be more likely to repeat the behavior. For instance, you might say, "Not eating red foods at school shows a lot of work; I like that." Or you could say, "I see that you are eating three meals every day and you are not snacking. You weren't doing that last week. I'm happy to see how you have changed your behavior. Good job!"

Other ways to express your pleasure and pride are with a smile, a wink, or a high-five. You might pat your son or daughter on the back, or squeeze his or her shoulder. Mary Ann Lucci found that she gave frequent hugs to her two daughters as they lost weight. "Sometimes when you say something to kids, they take it the wrong way and think that you're being sarcastic," she says, "so I would just hug my daughters when they did well."

Jan Richards occasionally stood up and cheered her nine-year-old stepson Thomas's behavior when he lost another pound — a gesture that always made Thomas smile. Another family offered a round of applause to the person who ate the fewest number of red foods during the week. Whatever form of praise you decide to use, be sure to support your children's progress briefly and specifically.

• *Rule 2: Praise good behavior immediately; say how pleased you are as soon as you notice it.*
The child who keeps below 1,200 calories for the day has really done well. Positively reinforce such behavior right away: "I am pleased that you stayed within the calorie range today. You did a good job." Try to show your pleasure as soon as possible after your children have tallied their calorie intake for the day. Children need to be rewarded with praise soon after each accomplishment. That helps them remember to repeat the good behavior. If you wait too long to give praise, children are not as likely to associate their hard work with your praise. Too much time has passed for them to make the connection.

Other times to praise children on the Stoplight Diet are right after they weigh themselves each day and fill in their weight chart, when they say "No thank you" to red foods, and when they eat less at meals. You can praise them on the spot for writing their food record in a neat, legible hand, for choosing a food that helps balance their diet, or for completing the food habit chart without being reminded. You can tell them how proud you are that they did not request red foods while grocery shopping. Examples of good praise are, "I'm really glad that you weighed yourself today without being asked," or, "You were so careful about not eating too many red foods this week — it really makes me proud."

· *Rule 3: Be consistent in your praise.*

Always respond in the same way to a behavior; never praise your children for doing something once and then punish them the next time they do the same thing. For example, never yell at your son for eating ice cream one day, and then, a few days later, offer him ice cream as a reward for cleaning his room. That kind of inconsistency confuses children, whether it entails learning the rules of the Stoplight Diet or knowing family rules.

· *Rule 4: Give attention only for appropriate behavior.*

Children love attention. They will try to grab the spotlight any way they can — even if it means doing something wrong. And rare is the parent who has not been disappointed in a child who, at one time or another, failed to do homework, rake the yard, or clean the dishes after dinner. Like praise, criticism is a powerful teacher. The difference is that criticism never instructs children how to change their behavior — it only shows them what they have done wrong. They may end up feeling hurt, and may even associate negative feelings with the parent who criticized them.

One way to short-circuit this process is to avoid nagging, lecturing, or yelling. Children often repeat the behavior that garners attention from parents — whether it is bad behavior or good. If you can teach your children that their good behavior gets more attention than the bad, you will be on the road to having a very powerful parenting tool.

Steven Jenkins found that he often criticized his son for not getting enough exercise. "You're lazy, Seth," he frequently told him. "You will never lose weight by sitting around the house all the time. You need to go outside and run or play ball or ride your bike. What's the matter with you, anyway?"

Seth responded to these harangues by becoming more withdrawn. He would sulk in his room and lose himself in comic books. Neither father nor son enjoyed being around each other very much.

In our program, Steven learned that his negative comments were driving a wedge between himself and his son. He learned how to stop criticizing Seth and discovered how to start focusing his attention and praise on his son's good behavior. The tensions eased. Steven also learned that he could help motivate Seth by demonstrating positive behavior. Each night Steven took a walk before dinner and invited Seth along. Seth refused for a few nights, but Steven went anyway and he never criticized Seth for not going along. Within a week, Seth was joining his father on the nightly walks. The two of them began talking while they walked and shared their daily experiences. "We have a whole different relationship now," Steven says. "It's much better."

• *Rule 5: Lavish praise especially often at the beginning of the Stoplight Diet program — when new behaviors and habits are being learned.*

Support and encouragement will help sustain your children, particularly during the crucial, early weeks when they are learning the Stoplight Diet. For a minimum of two weeks — and for as long as six weeks — each time you see your children doing something right on the Stoplight Diet, praise their behavior. It will take them about that amount of time to form a new habit or fully learn a behavior such as recording what they eat every day or weighing themselves.

You and your spouse know your children better than anyone else does. Once it becomes apparent that a child really has learned a new habit, you should let your praise taper off over the next six weeks or so. The reason is this: Praise, like any motivator, will not be effective if it is used too often. With time, it becomes monotonous, and may even sound insincere if used too frequently. But do not stop praising your children altogether. Praise will help them maintain their new health habits.

The Stoplight Diet Contract

Now that you know some important hints for praising your children, we want to teach you another management technique for parents called *contracting*.

As your children learn about the Stoplight Diet and begin to maintain their new eating, exercising, and self-monitoring habits, you should use less and less praise. But your children still need goals to work toward, and this is where the idea of contracting comes in, starting in Week 3.

With a written contract — an agreement between you and each of your children — you will establish a system of rewards for good behavior on the Stoplight Diet. These rewards should be privileges or activities that you and your spouse feel comfortable offering. You might, for instance, offer to take your family to an amusement park as a reward for your son having filled out his habit book without being reminded. Perhaps your daughter wants to attend an ice-skating competition; allow her to do so if she consistently stays within the four-red-foods limit.

Whatever rewards you and your spouse decide upon, make sure that the activity or privilege is something that you can provide soon after your child has earned it. That way your child connects the reward with the work that went into earning it.

Many families in our program offered a range of rewards. For example, they suggested some short-term, smaller rewards that a child could earn within a day or several days and then offered a larger reward that he or she could strive for over a period of weeks. You might, for instance, strike a deal with your child to fill out daily habit charts for two weeks straight without being reminded and then move back bedtime by an hour on a weekend night.

A larger reward — perhaps going on a camping trip — could be offered as an incentive for the child who achieves a certain weight loss over a period of two or three weeks. But make sure that you also require that all aspects of the Stoplight Diet program are followed: during this time, the child must stay within the allotted calorie range, eat a balanced diet, record his or her food, weigh in each day, and so on.

We suggest that you refrain from offering food, money, large gifts, or activities that occur too far in the future as rewards. Small rewards that can be earned weekly are best. We do not advocate giving money as a reward because we have found that the amount quickly escalates, usually at a rate faster than most parents can keep up with. We think it is better to limit the rewards to experiences — preferably those that you would not do frequently. It is best if at least some of the rewards involve the whole family; then everyone has a stake in following the Stoplight Diet. This also helps eliminate competition between siblings. The idea is for you and your family to spend more time together.

Among the wide range of activities that you can offer your children as rewards are these:

· Staying up one hour later on a weekend night
· Having a friend stay overnight

- Going to a movie
- Attending a special sporting event, concert, or fair

The list of possible rewards is endless. Once you and your spouse have targeted a few rewards that you feel comfortable offering, the next step is to explain the process to your child. Here is where you draw up a special contract between you and your son or daughter. It is important to be very specific. Whatever you offer, make sure that the rules are clear and in writing, as they are in figure 3 (page 66), which shows a sample contract. (Appendix G provides a blank contract form for you to photocopy and fill in, and the companion children's chapter discusses contracts in more detail.) One of the fringe benefits of these contracts is that you build your child's understanding of promises and commitments. That is an important lesson for life.

Now that you understand the importance of praising and contracting, you are ready for this week's quiz. By the end of Week 3 on the Stoplight Diet, your children should be recording with ease what they eat every day and successfully limiting their calories to 1,200 a day. They have probably lost a pound or two, and they should be familiar with the red, yellow, and green categories of foods, and should know how to limit themselves to four or fewer red foods a week (always eaten outside the home). As they progress on the Stoplight Diet, your children move toward a lifetime of good health.

FEBRUARY 5
date

I, ___PAT ROBINS___, agree to provide ___JAN ROBINS___
parent's name   child's name

with the reward named below once the following conditions are met.

___JAN___ will _(1) FILL IN HER STOPLIGHT DIET DAILY FOOD CHART_
child's name   fill in requirement

CORRECTLY EACH NIGHT, (2) STAY WITHIN THE 900-1,200 CALORIE RANGE,

AND (3) WEIGH HERSELF AND FILL IN THE DAILY WEIGHT CHART EACH DAY

during the next _7 DAYS_. When _JAN_
time period   child's name

has successfully done this, I will provide _A PAJAMA PARTY FOR_
fill in specific reward

TWO OF HER FRIENDS ON THE FIRST WEEKEND AFTER

SHE HAS EARNED THIS PRIVILEGE

___Pat Robins___   ___Jan Robins___
parent's signature   child's signature

Figure 3   Sample Stoplight Diet Contract

Week 3 Quiz

Answer true or false:

1. Praise can motivate your child to try harder.
2. Praise should come before the good behavior.
3. Praise should be used infrequently when you are first trying to change a habit.
4. A good rule when using praise is to offer it often in the beginning and to let it taper off later.
5. In addition to praising with words, you can also do so with gestures or expressions.
6. When praising a child, you should always be specific about the behavior being complimented.
7. To avoid confusing your children, you must be consistent in your praise.

Larry Jones wants to praise his ten-year-old son Fred for adhering to the Stoplight Diet. In the following examples, please provide some positive statements about the described behavior that Larry might use to praise his son and thus encourage his continued participation in the Stoplight Diet program.

8. Fred weighed himself in the morning without being asked. ____

____

9. When he came home from school, Fred passed up the opportunity to snack, and waited instead to have dinner. ____

____

10. Fred wrote down everything he ate during the day in his food record book. ____

____

Answers

1. True
2. False
3. False
4. True
5. True
6. True
7. True

8. "Fred, I am very pleased that you weighed yourself this morning."
9. "I'm proud of you, Fred. You did not have a snack when you came home from school."
10. "Fred, you have done a good job completing your food record book today."

Week 4
Exercise
Your Options

Welcome to Week 4 of the Stoplight Diet. You and your family have been eating more healthfully for three weeks. In just seven short days, you will pass the one-month mark!

Like most of the families on the Stoplight Diet, your family is probably attuned to the program by Week 4. Your good-eating habits are no longer new habits. You may even feel as though you have been eating this way all your life.

What is still a pleasant surprise, however, is the bathroom scale. By now, its readings should be moving downward — an accomplishment that makes it fun to chart body weight each day. You will not see a sharp drop, because the Stoplight Diet is designed for gradual weight loss. By losing weight slowly, you and your children have time to learn how to change your eating and exercise habits. This will help to ensure that the pounds you lose stay off permanently.

If you are not trying to lose weight but are sticking with the Stoplight Diet to encourage your son or daughter, these last three weeks have benefited you too. You are learning how to eat more nutritiously. If you (or any other normal-weight family members) are losing weight on the diet, adjust calories accordingly. Calculate your total daily calories and add 100 calories a day to that number until your weight reaches a plateau. At that point, you will have figured out your new daily calorie count.

Your family now knows that obesity is the result of an energy imbalance. If you eat too many calories — or if you do not burn enough calories — you add on pounds. You also know how to eat the right amount of calories to lose weight and how to eat well-balanced, nutritious meals even though calories are limited. In fact, you already have the first part of the energy imbalance in check: how many calories you eat. The next step is to tackle the second part of this energy imbalance: how many calories you burn.

Physical activity burns calories. And as you know, to lose a single pound, your body must burn 3,500 of the calories that would otherwise be stored as fat. For example, let's consider Sharon, a thirty-five-year-old woman who weighs 125 pounds. Sharon's body normally burns 2,000 calories a day in the course of her usual activity. By limiting the calories she eats to 1,200 a day, Sharon is burning 800 calories more each day than she is eating. This means that during one week, she burns an excess of 5,600 calories (7 days times 800 calories a day). As a result, Sharon loses about 1.6 pounds (5,600 total calories divided by 3,500 calories per pound) just by staying within her calorie range on the Stoplight Diet.

Now consider what happens when Sharon adds minimal exercise to her dieting. Suppose she walks just 15 minutes every day at a moderately brisk pace of 4½ miles per hour. In those 15 minutes, Sharon will walk a little over a mile and her body will burn 84 extra calories each day as a result. Over a week, that adds up to an additional 588 calories. This may not seem like much, but over six weeks, Sharon's 15-minute daily walk will burn off 3,528 total calories — more than a whole pound in lost weight. Not a bad payback for 15 minutes of daily activity.

The more you exercise, the greater the benefits and the sooner you reap them. Exactly how many calories are burned during exercise depends on the type of physical activity performed, how long it lasts, and the weight of the person doing it. The more a person weighs, the greater the calorie expenditure. Thus, a 75-pound child who walks for 10 minutes (at a speed of 4½ miles an hour) burns 34 calories, while a 150-pound adult doing the same burns 67 calories. The bottom line is that exercise speeds up the weight loss that you and your children have begun by following the Stoplight Diet.

Losing weight is only one of the numerous benefits of exercise. Physical activity actually helps to get rid of body fat. Studies show that dieting without exercise does accomplish weight loss. But what dieting alone cannot seem to change is body composition. Add physical activity and more body fat is lost than by dieting alone.

Research also indicates that exercise has these benefits:

• Heightens mood and generally makes a person feel better. Some scientific evidence ties this mood change to the production during exercise of beta-endorphins — brain chemicals that have been shown to make people feel calmer, happier, and more relaxed.

• Stimulates body metabolism, which results in more calories being burned. Studies show that exercise resets the metabolic rate to a higher-than-usual level for at least several hours after exercise is completed.

• Helps control a variety of conditions, from aging to diabetes. Physical activity also raises blood levels of high-density lipoproteins — HDL, the protective type of cholesterol. Load-bearing exercises, such as walking and jogging, help diminish bone loss and thus cut the risk of developing the debilitating, degenerative bone disease called osteoporosis, which frequently strikes older women.

• Reduces fatigue, improves blood circulation throughout the body, and may even improve the quality of sleep. Physical activity gives you more vigor. It makes you stronger, helps to tone muscles, and allows daily activities to become easier so that you have more vitality.

For all these reasons, during this, Week 4 of the Stoplight Diet, regular daily exercise will become an important addition to your family's new regimen.

Beginning this week, you and your family each need to expend an extra 50 calories a day by exercising. To meet this requirement, you can perform any kind of physical activity that you like. But whatever exercise you and your family engage in must be *in addition* to the activities that are already part of your regular daily routine.

For example, a child who already works a newspaper route may not count the time spent walking or riding a bike while delivering papers as exercise for the Stoplight program. Similarly, the child who already walks back and forth to school each day will need to find a new, additional activity to meet our 50-calories-a-day requirement. The point is to increase physical activity, since the present amount of exercise in the child's life has not been enough to maintain normal body weight. To lose weight most effectively, your son or daughter is going to learn to increase physical activity while eating less.

Appendix H, "The Stoplight Diet Exercise Guide," lists various kinds of activities and how many calories they burn (based on body weight). You and your children can use this information to calculate which forms of exercise will meet the 50-calories-a-day requirement. You may wish to mix the types of exercise you do to match your preferences, athletic prowess, and time schedule.

In choosing forms of exercise, and in guiding your children in their choices, keep in mind two key things: availability and enjoyment. Playing tennis is an excellent physical activity. But if it is expensive to play, difficult to find a court, or requires commuting a fair distance, then the odds are that you will not be able to play very often. Swimming is another great exercise. But if the pool is only open during hours that are inconvenient for you, or if chlorine bothers your eyes and you really do not care much for swimming, chances are you will not follow through on this activity.

Scientific evidence suggests that sporadic, inconsistent exercise provides few health benefits and may even be dangerous. To reap the most rewards from physical activity, you must do it often. Most experts believe that exercising a minimum of three times per week is necessary for optimum fitness. This means that once-a-week gym classes, once-a-week tennis, or once-a-week visits to a health spa are not enough to increase fitness or to guarantee weight loss.

How then do you fit daily exercise into an already busy family life? Why, the answer is at your feet. You and your family can walk.

Walking is one of the best exercises around. It costs nothing, can be done virtually anywhere, during any season of the year, and requires only a pair of comfortable walking shoes or sneakers for equipment. And to most people's surprise, walking burns nearly as many calories mile for mile as jogging.

Perhaps the best benefit of walking is that you and your children can do it together. That may sound like a simple concept, but it goes a very long way in encouraging your children. If you are like most parents who have participated in our program, you will find that walking with your children offers some special moments together in an otherwise hectic modern life.

Bill Wheeler, a forty-five-year-old television producer, recalls one particular walk that he shared with his eleven-year-old son Jeff. Bill and Jeff were walking through the park during a crisp winter evening. The sky was clear and the stars shone especially brightly.

"Jeff looked up as we walked and started asking me about the various constellations," Bill relates. "I pointed out a few to him, and then we started talking about the planets, and the next thing I knew he was telling me about his secret desire to be an astronomer. We had talked many times before about what he wanted to be when he grew up, but that's something that he had never mentioned before. It was such a special conversation, and we might never have had it had we not been on the walk together."

Other parents find that their children eventually look forward to walking together. "In the beginning my stepson John sometimes didn't want to go for a walk," explains Susannah Hopkins, whose twelve-year-old stepson lost 15 pounds on the Stoplight Diet. "But as the time wore on, he really seemed to enjoy it. And now he asks me every morning what time we will be walking each day.

"We use the time to exercise, but it's also a chance to catch up on everything that has happened during the day. Often my husband and I go together with John. If one of us can't break away from work, the other will walk with him.

"What I find so surprising is that it never takes us that long to do these walks. We generally walk about two to three miles, unless it's a really busy day, and then we'll just do one mile. If we walk just one mile it takes us about fifteen minutes. If we go farther, we end up walking for about thirty minutes to three-quarters of an hour. But it's never that much time. And we've come to really enjoy the walks."

Walking is also a great equalizer; just about everyone can do it, regardless of age or fitness level. Walking is particularly good for the overweight or very obese child who may not be used to getting any exercise at all. And even if there is a blizzard outside or steamy 95-degree weather, it is still possible to find a place to walk.

When the weather turned inclement, Wallace Edwards and her daughters often drove to a nearby shopping mall to walk indoors. If you do not have a shopping mall nearby, you can also walk up and down stairs. If your schedule is a problem, it is possible to combine commuting time with exercise by walking to work or to school. If the distance between home and office is too far to walk, then drive partway and walk the rest. Some parents who participated in our program walked during their lunch hour. Others who commuted by bus or train got off a couple of stops early and walked the rest of the way to their homes or offices.

Wherever and whenever you walk, you can count on this versatile exercise offering many advantages. You do not need a partner to walk. You can walk year round. And walking is a safe exercise, one that's linked to very few athletic injuries.

Walking also fits another requirement of the Stoplight Diet. It is what we call *life-style exercise,* meaning a physical activity that can be incorporated into a person's daily life.

Just as the Stoplight Diet is designed to change your family's nutritional habits for good, the program is also geared to helping you and your family make exercise part of your everyday life — a goal advocated by the American Heart Association, the National Institutes of Health, and other prominent medical organizations.

Our research shows that families who incorporate a variety of these life-style exercises into their daily routine are the most successful at losing weight and at making exercise a permanent habit. We compared two groups on the Stoplight Diet: families who did aerobic exercises only versus families who did a combination of life-style exercises. Two months into the program, both groups had lost about the same amount of weight. But at six months and again at eighteen months, the families who incorporated life-style exercises into their daily activities kept the weight off much better than the families who did only aerobic exercise. It seems that families whose exercise programs required special equipment were less successful at losing weight and at exercising regularly. The same was true of families who exercised at health spas, Y's, and other facilities that were not close to their homes or offices.

A program of life-style exercises incorporates all types of physical activity into a person's daily routine. And it does so in some very unexpected ways. It means using the stairs instead of riding the elevator. It means walking up or down escalators (rather than standing and letting them carry you to your destination). And it means using "foot power" whenever possible rather than riding in a car or other automotive vehicle.

Life-style exercise programs also include the more traditional physical activities, such as tennis, jogging, aerobic floor exercise, or karate. But unlike other exercise programs, life-style exercise does not depend on just these structured, scheduled activities. When your jogging partner is unavailable, when the weather turns bad, or when there is a hiatus in your aerobics classes, your exercise regimen will not come to a complete stop.

Here are some examples of the changes you can make to incorporate life-style exercises into your family's daily routine:

• Walk or ride a bicycle on short errands.
• Decrease your reliance on electrical appliances. That means using a hand beater instead of an electric one. Try a manual can opener instead of a motorized one. Hand-chop when possible instead of using an electric blender or food processor. Go back to a hand-powered toothbrush in-

stead of using an electric one. Stop using the remote control on the television, VCR, and stereo. Making such changes enables you to use more of your own energy.

• Stretch, walk, or otherwise move around instead of sitting and eating during a coffee break. Walk around the block before lunch.

• Remove extension phones where possible.

• Decrease the amount of time spent in sedentary activities, such as watching television or playing home video games. When you do watch television, combine it with a physical activity: ride a stationary bike or exercise during commercials. For example, a 150-pound person who jogs in place during the commercial breaks in a half-hour program burns an extra 50 calories.

We would like to offer some further advice about television — one of the major culprits behind inactivity. Everyone in your family may love watching television at some time or other. There is nothing wrong with that, but it is important not to let your television habits interfere with getting enough exercise. Here are some tips that will promote exercise:

• *Limit television viewing to evenings only — and preferably to just one hour.* Limiting television to evenings only — and to a certain number of hours or days of the week — encourages your children to exercise during the daylight hours after school. They can walk, jog, play a pickup game of basketball, or do something as simple as riding bicycles with their friends. Whatever they do, they are likely to get more exercise than they would sitting in front of the television set (and they will not be bombarded with food commercials). For the same reason, it is important to limit other sedentary activities, such as playing computer games. Encourage your children to be as active as possible. They will have more energy and be in better shape for their efforts.

You, of course, are an important role model. It is hard for children to understand limiting television viewing to an hour if you spend the entire evening glued to the set. Adhere to the hour limit yourself.

• *Move the television to a room in which the family spends little time.* Replace comfortable chairs in the television room with straight, hard-back ones that will reduce comfort and discourage television watching. Tie a ribbon around the on-off button on the television set to remind your children to do other activities rather than watch television. Do not keep the TV turned on for background noise or to entertain "company." When the television is on all the time (even when no one is watching it), it becomes easier for it to catch your attention and draw you into watching rather than doing something more active.

• *Keep a television log.* Do this for a few days. Watch television just as you normally do, but write down how many hours you spend viewing. We think you will be surprised at the result.

Making any or all of these changes puts you and your family on the road to incorporating life-style exercises into your daily routine. This means that regular physical activity is likely to become a permanent part of your lives.

You and your family can also plan more structured activities. One goal is to combine a program of aerobics and calisthenics. Aerobic exercises are those that burn a lot of calories and stimulate the heart and lungs to work harder. Calisthenics are exercises that do not burn a lot of calories but do reshape a person's body.

Examples of aerobic exercises are brisk walking, jogging, running, bicycling, swimming, basketball, and soccer. Calisthenics include jumping jacks, sit-ups, push-ups, and leg lifts.

Whatever combination of exercises you and your children decide to do, it is important that you begin slowly. It is also a good idea to check with your doctor before starting this or any other type of physical-activity program.

Initially, you and your family will do a small amount of exercise every day. (Even minimal amounts of physical activity can speed up weight loss, decrease appetite, and improve sleep.) Over the next several weeks, we will ask you to increase the exercise gradually, as your family gets in better shape and is able to endure physical activity for longer periods. Remember, as the amount of physical activity increases, so too will the number of calories burned.

As you know, during this first week of exercise, everyone in your family needs to expend 50 additional calories a day through some form of exercise. Two weeks from now, starting in Week 6 of the Stoplight Diet, you will raise the number of extra calories burned through exercise to 75 a day. And two weeks after that, beginning in Week 8, you will start to do enough exercise to burn an additional 100 calories a day. This means that starting four weeks from today, you and your children will be performing enough exercise to burn an extra 700 calories a week.

WEEKLY EXERCISE GOALS ON THE STOPLIGHT DIET

Time Frame	Number of Extra Calories Burned per Day	Number of Extra Calories Burned per Week
Weeks 4 & 5	50	350 (or 1 meal)
Weeks 6 & 7	75	525 (or 1½ meals)
Week 8 & thereafter	100	700 (or 2 meals)

That is the calorie equivalent of about two meals. The table above summarizes these exercise goals.

Remember not to overdo exercise. Increase your endurance gradually and encourage your children to do the same. Overexertion often results in injury, and injury usually means that you must stop exercising for a while. It is far better to exercise a little every day than to exercise too much once or twice a week.

Monitoring How Much You Exercise

Just as you monitor what you eat and how much you weigh each day, you need to keep track of how much you exercise. One easy way to do this is to record your exercise daily in your habit book. Appendix I provides a blank form that can be photocopied and used for this purpose, and figure 4 shows what a correctly filled-in exercise chart looks like for someone who weighs 130 pounds. Once you start recording your exercise, you should review this data every night with your children, just as you review the daily food and weight records.

Contracts and Exercise

Beginning with Week 4, you should include exercise as part of your child's weekly contract. To earn a privilege, your child now will be required to do all of these things:

· Record all foods eaten.
· Stay within the daily calorie range.
· Eat no more than four red foods.
· Weigh in every day.
· Burn an extra 50 calories a day exercising.

Name <u>MARLO</u> Week Number <u>8</u>

Calorie Goal: <u>100</u> per day/<u>700</u> per week

Day	Date	Type of Exercise	Time Spent Exercising (in minutes)	Number of Extra Calories Burned
Monday	5/5	BASKETBALL	10	58
Tuesday	5/6	SWIMMING { BREASTSTROKE / BACKSTROKE / CRAWL	10 / 10 / 10	40 / 32 / 40 } 112
Wednesday	5/7	WALKING (BRISK)	20	112
Thursday	5/8	WALKING (BRISK)	20	112
Friday	5/9	WALKING (LEISURELY) / BASKETBALL	20 / 10	60 / 58 } 118
Saturday	5/10	TENNIS	30	174
Sunday	5/11	WALKING (BRISK)	10	56
			Total	742

Figure 4   Sample Daily Exercise Chart

Your children will learn about this additional requirement in their Week 4 chapter on exercise, which also tells them that they will have to meet the terms of their contract for five out of the next seven days in order to earn their privilege.

In our program, some parents have reported that their children resist exercising even though it is required in a contract. To remedy this situation, we recommend that you exercise with your child whenever possible (as mentioned earlier). Try to set aside a regular time for exercising every day. If your child refuses to accompany you on a daily walk, go anyway by yourself. Each day, ask your child to go with you. If he or she refuses, do not yell or nag. Simply stick with your exercise regimen. We have found that most children will accompany their parents after a few days.

Of course, if your child refuses to exercise for more than a day or two, he or she will not earn the weekly privilege.

Week 4 Quiz

1. A program that incorporates increased physical activity into a person's everyday routine is called a _____ exercise program.

2. Which of the following statements are true?

    a. Exercise helps the body burn more calories.

    b. Physical activity specifically promotes the storage of body fat.

    c. Exercise improves blood circulation.

    d. Physical activity generally makes a person feel better.

    e. Exercise seems to raise blood levels of high-density lipoproteins, which helps protect against heart disease.

    f. You can never get too much exercise.

    g. Jogging burns calories at a much faster rate than walking does.

    h. No matter how much you exercise, you cannot burn more than 50 extra calories.

    i. It is best to use your car even on short errands so that you conserve energy for when you exercise.

3. A weight control program needs to include _____ as well as dieting to be really successful.

4. When choosing physical activities, it is important to keep in mind availability and _____.

5. One of the best forms of life-style exercise is _____.

6. Inactivity often stems from watching too much _____.

Answers

1. life-style	3. exercise	5. walking
2. a, c, d, e	4. enjoyment	6. television

Week 5
Setting
a Good
Example

As you open this chapter, your family begins the second month of the Stoplight Diet. They now know how to eat nutritiously and you have added exercise to their new life-style.

This week you will probably breeze through the grocery store, confident that you are able to choose yellow and green foods automatically. Red foods truly belong to the past during this, the fifth week of the Stoplight Diet.

"I still have a weakness for pastries," admits Barry Gregg, a thirty-two-year-old, barrel-chested father who lost 30 pounds on the Stoplight Diet in part by giving up the half dozen doughnuts and sweet rolls he used to consume on his nightly route as a distributor for a Pittsburgh newspaper. "I've learned to savor soda crackers instead."

The Greggs have made other changes as well. "We're very conscious of everything we eat now," says his wife, Linda, who trimmed 60 pounds off her five-foot-five-inch frame. "I don't fry foods anymore. In fact, if I look at greasy, fried foods, it makes me feel nauseous."

Another change the Greggs have made is in how they serve food. "We used to put platters of food on the table at dinner," explains Barry. "Now we measure and serve the food in the kitchen and then bring it to the table."

The Gregg family has also replaced white bread with fiber-rich whole-grain loaves. There is no more eating in front of the television and no reading the newspaper at the dinner table. They learned that if you eat in front of the television, each time you turn on the set you will think about eating again. Psychologically, you begin to pair watching television with eating. The same is true of reading the newspaper. If you eat something every time you open the paper, you will associate eating with reading. We have found that these are important habits to break.

"We don't enjoy eating out at fast-food places as much as we used to," says Linda, "because we find we can buy better food, prepare it at home, and enjoy it more."

The changes have paid off not just for Linda and Barry, who have battled weight problems all their lives, but for their six-year-old daughter, Sarah — the person who prompted their interest in the Stoplight Diet. Although her older brother, Hank, has always been very slim, Sarah showed clear signs of following in her parents' footsteps. At age five, she was a shy, round-faced child who carried 10 pounds of extra fat on her tiny body. Today, with her parents' help, Sarah is 10 pounds lighter — a loss that puts her back to the average weight for her height and age.

"Sarah has much more energy now," says Barry. "She laughs a lot more. She smiles more. She's much more outgoing. It's been quite a change for her."

Like the Greggs, your family is well on the way to achieving significant changes that contribute to a healthier way of living. In this second month of the diet, you may find that the program is slightly monotonous. Studies show that when people find food monotonous, they eat less — certainly a bonus for anyone who is trying to lose weight. But we do not want you to become bored with what you eat. It is certainly possible to eat healthfully and to eat interesting food. This is a good time to become more daring with new combinations of yellow and green foods. Take your children along as you explore the corners of your grocery store. Investigate new foods. Exotic fruits, such as papayas and cherimoyas (a custardlike tropical fruit), are now showing up in many American supermarkets. Use more spices and herbs, such as curry powder, cumin, and chili paste, condiments that can add zip to a stir-fried meal or liven up a low-calorie sauce. You might also try some of the new varieties of pasta available, including many from the Far East.

One family who stopped eating fattening desserts on the Stoplight Diet program rediscovered an old favorite — graham crackers. Other families have delved into ethnic cooking, experimenting with Indian, Chinese, and Middle Eastern dishes. Cynthia Reynolds and her daughters found a bakery that specialized in fresh, hot bagels. Tina Roberts

occasionally drove a few extra miles to splurge on fresh-picked rasp-
berries. "Compared to the fattening foods we used to buy, they were a
bargain," she says.

If you are like most families on the Stoplight Diet, this careful attention to good food choices is paying off with thinner figures and changing
appetites — all sure signs of the nutritional consciousness-raising that
is going on. And since your family is exercising every day, you may
notice an improvement in their physical condition. "We used to be tired
and out of breath all the time," says Linda Gregg. "But now that we
walk every day, we have a lot more energy."

Perhaps you are among the parents who report that their children are
now sleeping better. Maybe you are also noticing changes in your children's self-esteem. As their bodies become slimmer, their confidence
often grows. This is a good time to invest in a full-length mirror if you
do not already have one. Show your children how good they look.
Compliment them on their efforts. One family in the Stoplight Diet
program invested in a Polaroid camera and took pictures each morning
before school to bolster the children's sense of body image. In all likelihood, other people are beginning to notice the change as well. Your
children's friends, teachers, neighbors, and relatives may have started
to compliment them on their slimmer physiques.

You may also start to detect new social support for the changes your
family is making. When people understand how committed you and
your children are to achieving your goals, they often pitch in to help.
Mary Ann Lucci recalls how the mother of one of her daughter's friends
called to check the menu for an upcoming children's birthday party.
"Her son had told her that Anna was on a diet and so she called to
check what foods Anna could eat. I asked her to make sure that there
would be some diet sodas for Anna to drink, and then, the week of the
party, Anna ate no red foods in anticipation of eating a piece of birthday
cake at the party. It worked out very well."

How you and your spouse handle the various challenges that arise as
your family continues to follow the Stoplight Diet will help determine
the success your children have with the program. No family on the
Stoplight Diet lives in a vacuum.

Modeling

As a parent, you know already how impressionable children are. Like
most parents, you also are aware that children learn a large part of their

behavior by observing and imitating the people around them. Who are the people they are most likely to observe and imitate? You, their parents — the people they love and respect most.

It is common for children to follow the example of their parents almost too literally. Perhaps you have overheard your daughter in a make-believe play session with her dolls. There she was, reprimanding her "children" in the same tone and with the exact words that you use to correct her behavior. Or maybe you caught your son refusing to eat a food and uttering the same words that your husband uses to turn down the same dish.

Psychologists have a term for this normal act of learning by observation and imitation. They call it *modeling*. We all learn by modeling our behavior after the patterns of our parents, whether we realize it or not. Religious beliefs, cultural values, speaking style, and family rituals are passed from generation to generation through modeling.

One of the ways that children are likely to pattern themselves after their parents is in eating and exercise habits. The Stoplight Diet is designed to take advantage of this fact — for if children learn bad habits through modeling, they can learn good habits the same way. Parents who do best on the Stoplight Diet have children who do the best as well.

Parent Weight and Child Obesity

Scientists researching obesity have uncovered an important fact in recent years: how much a child weighs seems to be at least partly determined by how much the child's parents weigh. Are children overweight because their parents are? Is obesity passed through the genes the way parents pass on hair and eye color? Or is it simply the environment overweight children are reared in? Are they overweight because their overweight parents feed them fattening foods?

The answer to these questions seems to be that both nature *and* environment — or how parents rear their children — play a role in determining whether a child will be overweight or thin. Evidence of the role genes play in obesity comes from a study published in 1986 by Dr. Albert J. Stunkard. Dr. Stunkard reported on some four thousand pairs of twins in the United States and found that identical twins — those with the same genetic makeup — are more likely than nonidentical twins to show the same degree of obesity. In short, he found that genes, which determine a child's hair color and eye color, and which influence height and a host of other physical characteristics, also have a strong influence on childhood obesity. This does not mean that children with obese parents are destined to be obese themselves and should therefore give up all thoughts of dieting. What these findings show, says Dr. Stunkard, "is how important it is to start children who are at high risk for obesity on an early regimen of good nutrition and exercise" — precisely what the Stoplight Diet offers.

Our own studies show clearly that the success of children in losing weight is directly related to their parents' encouragement and to the involvement of their parents in the Stoplight Diet program. Children who do the best on the Stoplight Diet have parents who adhere to the program, who stay within the allotted calorie amounts, who provide well-balanced meals that are consistent with the requirements of the Basic Four food groups, who weigh in each day and record everything they eat, and who exercise daily to burn the necessary amount of calories.

The Stoplight Diet Starts with Parents

What these studies show is the importance of modeling. Your children watch and imitate your behavior all the time. If you overeat and fail to exercise, they will follow suit. But if you exercise regularly and eat well-balanced meals made up of nutritious foods, they will imitate that behavior as well.

How you follow the Stoplight Diet program is going to determine how well your children succeed at losing weight. Since you are their most important role model, you can teach them new habits through your own good behavior. If you do the things that you want them to do, they will learn to follow your lead. Each time you measure portions, or fill out the food record form, or turn down a red food, or chart your weight, you are showing your children a healthful new way of living. Each time you take a walk or play a game of tennis or climb a flight of stairs instead of taking the elevator, you make a statement about adhering to the lifestyle exercise requirements of the Stoplight Diet. And each time you slip up a little when facing a difficult situation, you can show them that no one is perfect, that everyone — including yourself — has to work hard to make changes in daily habits. Here are some suggestions for setting a good example for your children:

· *Call your children's attention to your good behavior.* This is the way you teach them how to improve their eating and exercise habits. Do not be afraid to instruct your sons and daughters in better health behavior. For instance, if you usually have cake for dessert every night but then learn to stop, point out the change to your children. Say to them: "Do you realize I am no longer eating cake for dessert? I am really enjoying this fruit."

Showing your children how to behave and then describing what you have done helps to reinforce the lesson they are learning. For example, the best way to get your son to record without delay what he has eaten for dinner is to sit down immediately after dinner and record what you yourself have eaten. Your son will then model his behavior after yours.

Susannah Hopkins, whose stepson, John, has successfully controlled his weight problem through the Stoplight Diet, makes a point of sitting near John when they go out to eat or to a party. In the beginning weeks of the Stoplight program, Susannah also tucked a copy of the food reference guide in her purse. At one pro hockey game, she and John walked from concession stand to concession stand to compare the choices. Then they consulted "The Stoplight Diet Food Guide" while standing in line. Among the choices for dinner were cheese nachos, hot dogs, pizza, and fried chicken. Drinks were limited to sugar-sweetened soft drinks, diet sodas, and beer. Susannah set a good example. She and John each ate one slice of pizza and drank a diet soda — both choices that are consistent with the Stoplight Diet. "But the best part was that neither one of us felt deprived," Susannah says. "We went to the game and we ate there by choosing wisely."

Susannah also consults with her stepson at restaurants. One of the family's favorite eating establishments specializes in seafood — although many of the dishes are fried, and french-fried potatoes come as an unrequested side dish. "The first time we went there, John was really disappointed about not being allowed to eat the french fries," Susannah says. "But he noticed that I ordered a baked potato. The next time we went, I reminded him that he could have a baked potato instead of the french fries and he was really pleased."

· *Praise your children when they imitate your good health habits.* This will reinforce their behavior. If you order a salad at a fast-food restaurant and your daughter then does the same (even though she loves greasy hamburgers), give her a hug or briefly comment on her smart choice. Praise as well the son who gets on the scale every morning, right after you do, or the daughter who burns 50 extra calories by joining in your daily family walk. As you have learned, praise works wonders in motivating children and is particularly effective when you combine it with modeling.

• *Convey a good attitude toward the Stoplight Diet.* Sometimes dieting is difficult and exercise is a bore. But parents who talk about how much they hate dieting or dislike exercise are likely to pass that message on to their children. If you need to vent your feelings, share them with your spouse or a friend at a time when your children are safely out of hearing range. Children quickly pick up — and model — the attitudes of their parents. Without realizing it, you can easily sabotage their good feelings for the program.

But do not hesitate to share some of the challenges you face. If you attend an office party and the only edibles in sight are all clearly red foods, explain to your children how you coped with the dilemma. Tell them how you asked for sparkling water with a twist of lime instead of an alcoholic beverage. Or explain how you slowly nibbled on only two of the cocktail-size fried egg rolls while your colleagues ate three times as many. Then record the red foods on your daily food record in front of your children. Share your experiences, but promote a positive attitude toward the program.

• *Call attention to your preferences for green and yellow foods.* When you choose low-calorie snacks such as fruits and vegetables, point out to your children that you have done so. Remind them that the family now snacking on popcorn instead of potato chips and dip. Occasionally take your children to the grocery store and take along this book. Have them help you pick out yellow and green food choices for the family.

• *Say "No thank you" to red foods when your children are present.* Children simply cannot understand why they are not allowed to eat something that you can eat. The often-quoted adage "Do what I say, not what I do" simply does not work on the Stoplight Diet.

If you must eat a red food in your child's presence, make sure that you eat it outside the home and do a quick tally to assure your son or daughter that you are not going beyond the maximum limit of four red foods a week. Also show your children that you have duly written down the red food on your food record sheet, and be prepared to offer them the same red food that you are eating or a suitable substitute.

• *Exercise with your children whenever possible.* There is no better way to encourage them to get more physical activity than to exercise with them. Walk. Ride a bicycle. Play a game of tennis. Shoot some baskets.

Do whatever you like, but do some kind of exercise with them and try to make it a daily event.

· *Keep good daily food records as an example to your children.* The more they realize that you are all in this together, the better they will do on the Stoplight Diet. Each time you write down what you have eaten during the day, they are reminded to do the same. If you record your food right after a meal, chances are that they will follow suit.

· *Practice table manners that suit the Stoplight Diet.* Modeling is a slow process, but it pays off with big dividends. Eat slowly. Take small bites and chew your food slowly. Another trick is to put your fork down between each bite; do not pick it up again until you have finished swallowing. Disband the "Clean Plate Club." Instead, encourage your children to eat only until they feel full (as long as they eat nutritiously).

· *Teach your children how to overcome occasional lapses.* If you have a bad day and slip off the Stoplight Diet, it is okay to share that news with your children. They need to know that it is not the end of the world to go over the calorie limits. But also explain the circumstances and tell them how you will prevent subsequent lapses. Make sure that a bad day does not become a habit, and use it to teach your children about self-tolerance — a lesson they can apply to all aspects of their lives.

· *Be the model for patience and perseverance.* Show your children that you are not giving up, even when your weight hits a plateau. We encourage you to talk about your disappointment when this happens. Share your feelings with your children. Tell them how you know that if you wait until next week, you will probably lose a pound. By discussing these issues, you will teach them that although changing health habits takes determination, it is ultimately worth the effort.

Be patient. Changing behavior is a slow process. No one changes in a day or a week. Even if you did change that quickly, in all likelihood the change would not be permanent. If some days seem harder than others, do not be discouraged. Keep modeling and praising, modeling and praising, modeling and praising. You might also take heart from the example of the four-member Bernhardt family, which lost a total of 150 pounds on the Stoplight Diet and, most important, is still keeping the weight off more than two years later. "Some days it was hard," notes Celia Bernhardt. "We were changing so many things in our lives. And there would be weeks when it seemed like it was one step forward and two steps backward."

But the hard work did pay off, Celia says, reaching inside her purse for the wallet-size snapshots of her daughters before they lost weight. One photo shows seven-year-old Karen as an unsmiling, obese little girl, looking as though she has been stuffed into the too-tight plaid dress she is wearing. The second photograph shows Amelia, almost as obese as her younger sister. Unlike Karen, Amelia is smiling; but in doing so, she reveals the folds of a double chin.

Both photographs are hard to reconcile with the two slim girls Celia's daughters have become. Amelia has long, lean legs that she likes to show off in designer jeans. Her double chin is gone, but she still flashes a broad smile. Like her sister, Karen also has a reason to smile. "Since I lost ten pounds on the Stoplight Diet, I've made a lot more friends. Now it's fun to ride a bike or play softball with them because I don't get out of breath anymore."

In this chapter you have learned the importance of setting a good example for your children. The more you can be a model of good behavior for them to follow on the Stoplight Diet, the better they will succeed in their quest to exercise more, eat more nutritiously, and lose weight.

The following quiz, like the others, will help you review what you have learned. Remember to look back and reread pertinent sections of the text if you have difficulty on the quiz. If you are passing the book on to your spouse, use a separate sheet of paper to record your answers. When you are finished, give the book to your children so that they can read the companion chapter, which is also about setting a good example. And be sure to review the chapter with them and assist with their quiz. Do not be surprised if they try to set a good example for you!

Week 5 Quiz

1. When children observe and imitate the eating habits of their parents, they are exhibiting the type of behavior that psychologists call _____.

2. Parents who try to change their children's behavior by setting a good example are using _____.

3. Research shows that obese parents often have _____ children.

4. To lose weight, people must change their _____ habits and their _____ habits.

5. To set a good example for your children, it is important never to eat foods from the _____ color group in front of your children.

6. Which of the following actions are ways to set a good example for your children on the Stoplight Diet?

    a. Limiting red foods
    b. Exercising daily
    c. Eating ice cream in front of your children
    d. Recording what you eat each day
    e. Telling your children what you weigh every day

7. When your children follow the good example you are setting on the Stoplight Diet, it is important to _____ them for their efforts.

Answers

1. modeling
2. modeling
3. obese

4. eating/exercise
5. red

6. a, b, d, e
7. praise

Week 6
Making
New Rules

For the past five weeks, you and your family have been engaging in some significant alterations in life-style. You have learned much about exercise, nutrition, weight loss, and new parenting techniques. By setting a good example, you are teaching your children a lesson about self-control and motivation that will serve them well whether they apply it to losing pounds or working harder in school.

You have been your children's teammate in the Stoplight Diet program. You have cheered them on through the lessons about red, yellow, and green foods, through the early days of logging what they eat and keeping track of daily weight. You have been a good model, by showing your child how to eat and exercise in a new way.

As a parent, you are, of course, more than just a teammate. You are also a coach. Coaches set rules for their team. They must provide discipline, monitoring, and motivation. You must do the same on the Stoplight Diet for your child to succeed.

Your new skills now give you many more options to help shape your children's behavior, whether it is changing what they eat or when they go to bed. You now know how to motivate your children — an important skill that many parents never master. This week, we thought it would be helpful to expand on what you have learned. The following discussion draws upon some of the principles you now know and suggests new ones to apply when making new rules.

- *Observe your child closely before instituting a new rule.* Determine if an unwanted behavior occurs frequently enough to warrant changing.

There should be no ambiguity about whether a behavior is appropriate or inappropriate. For instance, if you think that your daughter is snacking, observe her behavior for a week. Keep a written record of how many times you see her snacking. Is it just one or two nights that she has an apple before dinner, or is it most evenings? You can make the determination by watching carefully before you say anything to your daughter.

• *Institute only one new rule at a time.* Changing more than one behavior is confusing and difficult for a child. Recognize that forming a new habit is a slow process. This is why we introduce new ideas each week, rather than all at once. It would be too difficult, for example, for a child to learn all the Stoplight Diet food rules, start exercising, and begin adhering to contracts all in the same week. By spreading these lessons over several weeks, you give your child a chance to learn each of them fully.

• *Make the rule specific.* Carefully-thought-out rules stipulate a behavior and a consequence. Simply telling your son to "complete your food record for today" does not tell him much about what will happen if he does — or if he does not — do what you have requested. But if you say, "When you've finished filling out your food record for today, I will play catch with you for ten minutes," your son has an incentive to complete the task. Younger children, those aged six and seven, respond especially well to small, daily goals set by their parents. Unlike their older siblings, it is hard for them to grasp the idea of working toward goals that are too far in the future for them to really understand.

There are also no incentives attached to the directive "Don't eat red foods." Imagine saying this instead: "If you do not eat any red foods all day, I will play one computer game with you before bedtime."

• *State the rule in a positive way.* Everyone responds better to positive statements than to negative ones. Children are no exception. Try to keep rules short and to the point. Rather than threatening your children with, "You can't go to the zoo if you don't exercise," remind them with, "Exercise before you go to the zoo." It makes the choice for them easy and more appealing. They will also get the message that they are being allowed to watch television as a reward for exercising, rather than being penalized for not exercising. This is a subtle but very important difference.

Here is another example of communicating a rule in the affirmative: Instead of saying, "You're not allowed to turn on the stereo and listen to your favorite song while you get dressed unless you weigh yourself first before breakfast," you could deliver the same message with, "If you weigh yourself before breakfast, then you may listen to your favorite song on the stereo while you get dressed." Notice that the emphasis again is primarily on the behavior you want your child to follow — and secondarily on the reward it will bring them.

• *Set a reasonable rule — one that is within your child's mental and physical abilities.* Improvement comes in small steps. It is unrealistic to expect changes overnight. If you establish unrealistic goals, you will only set up your children for frustration and disappointment. It would be unfair, for instance, to expect a child to walk 2 miles in 20 minutes. When you say to your daughter, "If you walk two miles in twenty minutes, you may stay up an extra half an hour," both of you know there is little chance that she will be able to accomplish that goal. But if you say, "Walk two miles in *forty* minutes and you may stay up an extra half an hour," you set a reasonable goal — one that could gradually increase her walking speed.

It is also important to keep in mind your child's mental capabilities when setting rules. A child who suffers from learning disabilities will probably have trouble recording food each day and tallying calories. You will need to help. But give your son or daughter as much control over these tasks as is feasible for his or her capabilities. This will heighten the child's sense of self-control.

• *Set a rule that is enforceable.* It makes no sense to set a rule if you cannot see that it is carried out. The child who eats dinner each night alone is probably going to have trouble adhering to the Stoplight Diet principles. So is the child whose parent is too busy to review the food record form and too preoccupied to look over the exercise log. For your child to succeed, you need to be there to participate, to provide support, and to enforce rules. Can you imagine how a team of athletes would fare if its coach rarely attended practice?

Remember that you now have a whole new array of parenting tools. They are all you need to help change your children's eating and exercise behavior. As you employ these new tools, you will see how powerful they are in promoting good health behavior for your children.

There is also a bonus. As mentioned, the techniques that you have learned on the Stoplight Diet to help your children lose weight can also be used to change other behaviors. For instance, are you tired of having to struggle to have your children come home on time for dinner? Would you like them to do their homework without prodding? Or to clean

TIPS ON COMMUNICATING NEW RULES

• Define the new rule. (For example, "You must fill out your Stoplight Diet food record form by eight o'clock each night.")
• Determine the privilege your children will receive for following the new rule, and be specific. (For example, "If you do this every night this week without being reminded, you will be allowed to stay up an extra half hour on Friday and Saturday nights.")
• Word the rule in a positive way. ("If you fill out your food record form each night this week by eight o'clock without being reminded, you may stay up an extra half hour on Friday and Saturday nights.")
• Draw up a weekly contract that includes the new rule. Remember to be very specific. You may want to give your children a little leeway by requiring they observe the new rule for only five out of the next seven days. That way they will not give up if they forget to adhere to the rule early in the week.
• Post the rule in an obvious place. It will serve as a good reminder for your children. You can even enlist their help in making a sign and choosing where it should be placed.

their rooms regularly without a fight? Try writing a contract to encourage the desired behaviors, but keep in mind one very important caveat: Never mix Stoplight Diet contracts with contracts designed to change other behaviors. The two types should always be independent. Make sure your children understand that changing how they eat and how they exercise has nothing to do with contracts about how well they keep their rooms clean, how often they set the table for dinner, or whether they are home on time.

We have found that when parents mix these contracts, the tasks become overwhelming and their children receive confusing messages. Think of a child who did all that was required for the Stoplight Diet one week, but forgot to clean up his room. If his weekly contract required him to adhere to the Stoplight Diet as well as clean his room, he obviously has not earned his weekly privilege. This child will feel pretty discouraged, since all his good efforts on the Stoplight Diet were for naught. By having separate contracts, he can be rewarded for sticking with the

Stoplight Diet, but not for cleaning his room. That is as it should be, since they are very different behaviors.

Week 6 Quiz

Answer true or false:

1. It is not important to explain rules to children if they read the companion chapter of this book.
2. Before you set a new rule, it is necessary to observe your children's behavior.
3. It is best to change several types of behavior at the same time by setting several new rules.

Six-year-old Paul and his mother, Lori, were waiting in line at a fast-food restaurant.

"I want a hamburger, french fries, and a chocolate shake, Mom," said Paul.

Lori reminded him that french fries and a chocolate shake are red foods. "How many red foods have you eaten this week, Paul?"

Paul looked very glum. "I've had four, Mom," he said.

Lori told him to choose something else to drink and Paul began to cry very loudly. "Stop crying right now," she warned.

With that, Paul cried even louder. Lori suddenly felt embarrassed when she saw that everyone standing in line was beginning to stare.

"What'll it be today, ma'am?" the boy behind the counter asked her.

"Two hamburgers, french fries, and a chocolate milk shake," she said, thinking to herself, I'll give him what he wants just this one time.

Paul stopped crying.

Answer true or false:

4. Paul learns from this incident that crying gets him what he wants.
5. Paul is not likely to repeat this behavior.

6. In the future, which of the following actions could Lori take to best handle a situation like this?

   a. Prepare Paul before they go into the restaurant.
   b. Suggest green and yellow food alternatives.
   c. Ignore Paul's crying, and if it continues, instruct him to sit in the car.

    d. Yell at Paul to stop crying, and if that does not work, swat him once.

    e. Never stop at a fast-food restaurant again.

    f. Remind Paul of his contract not to eat more than four red foods a week.

Judith Gonzalez has explained the following rule to her eight-year-old daughter, Carla: Carla is not allowed to eat food from other people without checking with her mother first. Judith knows that Carla understands this rule, so she is surprised to look out the window one afternoon and see Carla licking a double-decker ice-cream cone.

"Where did you get the ice cream?" Judith asks her daughter.

"From Tony's mother," Carla replies.

7. Which of the following should Judith do?

    a. Take the ice cream away from Carla.

    b. Tell Carla that the ice cream counts as a red food for this week.

    c. Talk to Carla about learning to say "No thank you" to red foods.

    d. Speak with Tony's mother. Explain that the Gonzalez family is on the Stoplight Diet. In addition, tell her that Carla is not allowed to take food from other people without asking her mother first.

Answers

1. False   4. True   6. a, b, c, f

2. True   5. False   7. b, c, d

3. False

Week 7
On the Road
from Red
to Green

By this week of the Stoplight Diet, your family has changed its eating habits, initiated a regular program of exercise, and learned a great deal about nutrition. But as you well know, your family is still bombarded with temptations: television commercials extolling the delights of the latest fast food or the newest flavor of ice cream, appealing supermarket displays designed to challenge the strongest willpower, and restaurants offering lavish, high-fat, tempting dishes.

During the final weeks of the formal program at the University of Pittsburgh, every Stoplight Diet family learns how to deal with temptations. We call this part of the program *controlling your environment*. It will be one of your final lessons in the Stoplight Diet program.

Everyday Cue Control

Psychologists have a term for the way certain signals help to produce a particular behavior: *cue control*. There are cues for feeling sleepy, cues for physical activity, and cues for eating.

Hunger is one example of a cue for eating. It is an internal cue, caused by physical changes in the body. When you do not eat for long periods, your blood sugar levels drop and start a cascade of reactions in your body that prompt hunger. You eat something and the hunger ends. Temperature can also work as an internal cue. When your body is cold, it sets off a response in the brain that prompts you to eat more and store extra fat. Similarly, sleep deprivation can be a cue for hunger.

There are many external cues — cues in the environment — that prompt hunger as well. Time of day is one of the chief environmental cues. If you are used to eating lunch at twelve-thirty every day, odds are that you will feel hungry at that time just by looking at the clock. Seeing food or smelling food can also prompt the desire to eat. Think of being in the middle of a bakery surrounded by glass cases of french pastries. Or how about catching a whiff of a Chinese restaurant during the height of the dinner hour? Few people could be in those situations without being tempted to eat.

Social pressures also provide important eating cues: seeing all the children on your block line up for the ice-cream truck, for instance, or attending a wedding with an open bar, numerous hors d'oeuvres, and a lavish sit-down dinner. All these various types of cues will prompt people to eat, whether or not they are physically hungry.

Studies show that overweight people often eat in response to external cues, even when they are not truly hungry. Many people also eat when they are stressed, anxious, or depressed. With a little training, however, it is possible to gain control over the numerous cues that control eating. Here is what we recommend:

• *If you or your children feel hungry in between meals, wait twenty minutes before eating anything.* While you are waiting, divert attention from food by doing something else. Drinking a glass of water is a good interim tactic. Usually after twenty minutes, you will find that your hunger is gone. *Remember that hunger goes away whether you eat or not.* If you must eat something, munch on carrot or celery sticks. They require a lot of chewing and are very filling. Other options include eating a rice cake or having a piece of fruit.

• *Reduce the times and situations where you eat.* Remember that when you cook, it is very easy to eat several hundred calories without realizing it. Next time you prepare a meal, see how many times you "sample" or "taste" what you are eating. Then add up the calories. You will be surprised at how much can be consumed when you are not thinking about it.

Eating in front of the television is another easy way to overeat, as you already know. So is eating with your nose stuck in a newspaper or your eyes glued to a book or magazine. Pay attention when you eat. Limit your eating to the kitchen and the dining room or the breakfast nook. The fewer places in your house devoted to eating, the fewer the hunger cues you and your family will feel.

• *Keep food stored out of sight.* Red foods are not allowed in the house, of course. Store yellow foods out of sight whenever possible. The fewer foods readily available, the less the temptation to eat. Also, avoid using those popular magnetic "food look-alikes" that often adorn refrigerator doors. If you use a cookie magnet to hold the shopping list, you are sending a subconscious food message to your family.

• *Serve measured portions from the kitchen. Avoid eating "family-style."* One of the goals of the Stoplight Diet is to teach yourself and your children how to eat less. You cannot do that if there are platters and bowls of food on the table. It is also difficult to measure what you and your family eat if you serve meals family-style. Serving from the kitchen means that you reduce the temptation to eat more than the food that is placed on your plate. Another hint is to serve portions on smaller plates to give the illusion that you are eating more.

• *Never skip meals.* People who diet often cut back on the number of times they eat during the day. That is a bad idea. They end up waiting so long to eat that their hunger is hard to control. By eating three meals a day, you will decrease snacking between meals and help guarantee that you and your children will not be tempted to overeat.

Just as cue controls help determine when your family eats, they also dictate when your family exercises. To help promote exercise and other activities, we recommend the following cue controls:

• *Keep reminders of physical activity in sight.* If exercise clothes, shoes, balls, and other equipment are easy to get at, they will be used more often. Purchase sports magazines as reminders of various types of exercise.

• *Try to set a regular time for exercise every day.* While you are engaging in many life-style exercises, such as using the stairs instead of riding the elevator, it is also important to have a routine for regular exercise. If you take a walk every day before dinner, you will be reminded that it is time to go exercise when that hour rolls around.

Special Times

With almost two months of the Stoplight Diet behind you, you and your family clearly can handle most everyday situations. But some of the most difficult situations you will face involve special occasions — birthdays, Christmas, Hanukkah, family reunions, anniversaries, weddings, bar mitzvahs, Halloween, Easter, Thanksgiving, school and office parties — which can strain anyone's willpower.

There is no question that these special occasions can be challenging for people who are dieting or changing the way they eat. But like learning which hunger and exercise cues to pay attention to — and which ones to ignore — handling the special occasions that face all of us numerous times during the year is also possible.

One of the first steps we recommend is adding up the various special occasions that your family celebrates yearly. In addition to those already mentioned, include other religious events and national holidays. When you add up the various occasions during the year, you will find that your family celebrates at least one special occasion a month, perhaps more.

Everyone likes to celebrate. Certainly these holidays are a time to break loose and indulge yourself a little bit. But when you realize how often such occasions occur, you can see that it is important to exert some restraint.

• *Plan ahead.* Whether it is Christmas, a birthday celebration, or just a slumber party for your children, planning is essential. If you know your family will be eating away from home and that there is likely to be a lot of food available, encourage them to eat a smaller breakfast and lunch that day. Help them plan their red foods for the week accordingly.

• *Limit celebrations to one per day.* If this sounds obvious, think of the times that you may have celebrated a birthday with different groups of people. Or consider the Christmas season, when there is often more than one party a day to attend.

• *When you entertain, cook only for the size crowd expected.* If you are worried about not having enough food, then cook a little extra, but be sure to send all fattening leftovers home with the guests.

• *Display good health habits for your children to model by not baking cakes, cookies, candies, fruit breads, or other high-calorie red foods.* If you must bake, consider making lower-calorie cookies, such as ginger snaps or homemade graham crackers. Bake whole-fiber breads and rolls. Focus on homemade pickles, mustards, and relishes rather than sugar-filled jams and jellies.

• *When you must offer a red food, limit the number of servings you prepare.* Few people can imagine celebrating a birthday without a cake and, usually, ice cream. Tradition is fine. But instead of baking a 9-inch layer cake to serve to a party of four, consider making individual cupcakes or baking a smaller cake. The point is to make no more than one serving of a red food per person. If you prepare more, give it away to guests or neighbors.

• *When invited to a friend's or relative's home for a holiday, offer to bring a low-calorie dish that your family and other guests can enjoy.* Our experience is that many guests are pleased to find one or two low-calorie dishes that they may enjoy with relative caloric impunity. You can help your family minimize calories by encouraging them to eat the low-calorie food you provide.

• *When possible, enlist the help of your hosts.* Tell your hosts that your family is trying to improve their health habits. Explain that they eat many types of foods, but that they limit consumption of high-calorie dishes. If appropriate, ask your hosts for help in curtailing how many red foods are served. It is also helpful to suggest some alternative items. Obviously, your request requires tact, and there will be some instances where it is not possible to make this request. The better you know your hosts, the easier it will be to ask for their assistance.

• *Start new family traditions.* Whenever possible, revamp activities that involve food. Instead of giving candy for Valentine's Day, give a long-stemmed rose. Rather than filling Easter baskets with chocolate-covered bunnies and jelly beans, provide toys, comic books, or stuffed animals. Other good treats are books, balloons, Silly Putty, crayons — in short, anything that does not entail food.

On birthdays, promote games and activities rather than food-related parties. You could take your children and their friends to a movie, a museum, or to an ice-skating rink. You might go on a bicycle ride and pack a nutritious picnic lunch. Or you could offer the birthday celebrant an overnight camping trip that includes a long hike.

• *At family celebrations, plan activities that will minimize the time spent around the dining-room table.* Clear the table as soon as eating is finished. Lingering at the dinner table means that more food will be consumed. Move everyone to another room as soon as possible after the meal is finished. Play games, show home movies, sing and play the piano, have older family members regale the younger relatives with a night of oral history. Make a home video movie. Go for a walk. In other words, do anything that is unrelated to food or eating.

• *Practice smart party tactics: do not sit or stand near the food if possible.* Teach your children to do the same by helping them plan ahead for parties. Gently — and privately — remind your children at parties to slow down if you find them gorging on food. Nurse one or two low-calorie beverages. (We know many people who stay slim by bringing their own low-calorie beverages.) Practice saying "No thank you," and encourage your family to follow your example.

• *No matter what you eat at a party, never take high-calorie leftovers home.* Bringing food home guarantees that you will eat it.

• *Before eating out, help your children plan what they will order.* Begin by choosing a restaurant that offers low-calorie foods. Seafood restaurants are a good choice, provided they offer food that is broiled, baked, or grilled rather than deep-fried. Ethnic restaurants often can be a good choice. Find an Italian restaurant that specializes in spaghetti and good vegetable dishes, or a Chinese restaurant that makes spectacular whole fish with black-bean sauce or some other specialty. Careful calorie choices can also be made easily in Japanese restaurants, Middle Eastern restaurants, and even pizza parlors.

Before you go to the restaurant, discuss with your children what they want to order. Preplanning helps them make better choices later. Remember to be a good role model in what you order as well.

• *Plan ahead for vacation eating.* Avoid making vacations a license to overeat. Keep busy during vacations. The more non-food-related activities you help your family engage in, the less time you will have to eat. When possible, bring along low-calorie snacks (carrot sticks, fruit, diet soft drinks, jugs of ice water), whether it is for a long car trip or a visit to the zoo. By all means, try new restaurants while on vacation, but keep in mind low-calorie, low-fat choices. It makes no sense to blow months of hard work during two weeks of relaxation.

Building a Support System

Relatives

Some of the families in our Stoplight Diet program found great support when they told their relatives they were embarking on a weight-loss plan. In many cases, they discovered that their added pounds had been a source of concern for the relatives, who worried about their having a heart attack, developing obesity, or even getting cancer.

Other families, however, encountered a surprising amount of resistance, pressure, and guilt when they informed grandparents, aunts, and uncles of their new life-style. "You'll stunt your children's growth," was a common cry. "They'll grow out of it — it's just baby fat," was other frequently heard advice. "How can you do this to my grandchild!" lamented one concerned grandmother, who is obese herself.

Relatives may even engage in occasional sabotage. Beryl Marx found that her mother secretly tried to press candy on Beryl's daughters during their weekly visit. When Beryl confronted her mother and asked her to please stop giving the girls candy, she refused. One day she even managed to stuff a piece of candy in her youngest granddaughter's mouth. "Claire spit it out," Beryl says. "She knew better, even if my mother didn't. Fortunately, she's seen how serious we are about all this and she's stopped that behavior."

If you experience similar problems with your relatives, we recommend that you ignore their interference. If it continues, ask them to stop sabotaging your efforts. Instruct your children to be firm in their "No thank yous" to well-meaning yet unsupportive relatives. In some cases, you may have to limit their time together, or allow your children to visit only when you or your spouse can supervise. Prepare yourself for some tough conversations.

When Linda Gregg's aunt demanded, "What kind of life are you giving your children? You're not feeding them and they're not watching television," Linda confidently responded, "We're giving them a healthier life."

The Greggs also found that they had to prepare for family reunions, where, as Barry Gregg explains it, "everyone stuffed food in the kids." They cut back on the food their family ate the week before the reunion, and made sure that no red foods were consumed in the days immediately preceding the family gathering. They coached their children not to overeat. They discussed the kinds of foods that would be available and helped their children plan what they would eat.

"The only thing to do on those days is to minimize the damage as much as possible," says Linda.

Of course, not all relatives will sabotage the Stoplight Diet. Cynthia Reynolds recalls a Christmas party where her cousin, who's a physician, spotted her eating one too many cookies. He took her aside and said, "Stop that, Cynthia. You look so good now. I'm not going to let you get fat again."

Neighbors

You may not know it, but your neighbors often provide a lot of food for your children. "We never realized how much food our kids were getting from the people next door," says Bill Wilson.

The Wilsons discovered that well-meaning neighbors were baking special treats for their children and helping to contribute to their daugh-

Week 7: On the Road from Red to Green · 103

ter Sasha's growing problem with obesity. So when the Wilson family began the Stoplight Diet, they let their neighbors and their friends know about their new eating habits. They found a great deal of support. "Our next-door neighbors stopped baking cookies for the kids and started giving them pretzels and popcorn instead," says Bill.

Cynthia Reynolds and her family also sent out the word around the neighborhood. "At Halloween, people gave us fruit or pennies instead of candy," says Cynthia's daughter Connie. "They made it special just for us."

Blended Families

Blended families often face an additional challenge on the Stoplight Diet. Susannah Hopkins recalls how her husband's former wife not only refused to cooperate with the Stoplight Diet, but tried to sabotage it. "My stepson, John, visits his mother every other weekend. The rest of the time, he lives with us. So for two weeks, the family would work really hard on the Stoplight Diet, and John would lose weight. Then he would go to his mother's house and she would give him as many fattening foods as she could — Coke, cookies, fried foods, whole milk instead of skim, potato chips, and other types of junk foods. One weekend, John gained four pounds. It was very discouraging."

Although John's mother refused to help, Susannah and her husband, Dan, did not give up. They sent enough food record forms with John each weekend for his mother and stepfather to participate. They included a detailed description of the diet and they encouraged John to explain the rules of the Stoplight Diet to his mother. Nothing seemed to help. Then came one of the worst weekends. John had by then lost a total of 6 pounds. His mother called and promised him that she would make barbecued spareribs — one of his favorite foods — as a "reward" for losing weight. "John was terribly excited, until we explained that barbecued ribs are one of the most fattening foods you can eat," Susannah says. "We also reminded him that we don't reward weight loss with eating. He was very disappointed."

Dan recalls phoning his former wife and asking that she not make the spareribs. "I asked for more cooperation on the diet. She wouldn't agree, but at least she didn't go ahead with the ribs."

Susannah and Dan explained to John that he was getting old enough to take some of the responsibility for what he chose to eat — even when tempting red foods were around, and even when the person offering them was his mother. "We tried to role-play how he could say 'No thank you' to the foods his mother offered," Dan notes. "And we helped him think of good alternatives when faced with a lot of red foods."

Eventually, John's mother recognized his achievement, thanks to Susannah's and Dan's efforts. John's mother even wrote a note thanking them for helping him to slim down.

Not all blended families go through the kind of struggle the Hopkins family faced. But there is always extra coordination involved when children split their time between two households. If that is the case in your family, here are some suggestions:

• Ask for special help from the noncustodial parent. Explain the Stoplight Diet (or present a copy of this book) and tell the other parent how important *every* family member's participation is to the success of your child.

• Assure the noncustodial parent that he or she does not have to try to lose weight to participate in the Stoplight program, but that your child does need his or her support and encouragement.

• Teach your children that the Stoplight Diet applies no matter which household they are in. Explain that it is up to them to make choices about food — and that sometimes those choices will be difficult.

• Siblings can also be a source of support. In the Hopkins family, John's older brother Wyatt offered aid when the boys were at their mother's house. "He kept a log of his food even though he didn't need to lose weight and he asked his mother to please help John more," Susannah says.

School Personnel and Teachers

Your children eat approximately five meals a week at school. If you are lucky, you may be able to pack a lunch each day and in this way control what they are eating. But if you are like most parents, your children probably eat a significant number of lunches prepared in the school cafeteria.

For this reason, we recommend that you enlist the help of school personnel and teachers. You may need to have a special meeting with your child's adviser or the principal. If the school does not provide skim milk at lunch, ask that it be made available. Many schools will not be able to offer special meals, but you can ask that your children be allowed to make several selections from the salad bar on the days when fried entrees or other fattening foods are served. Soup made without cream is also a good low-calorie substitute for high-calorie foods.

We have found that most school personnel are supportive of the Stoplight Diet program. When the Drummonds found that their son's school required that students eat lunch family-style, they requested that their son be allowed to choose his food from the school's salad bar on days when fattening meals were served. Their son, Tommy, filled his plate full of salad, hard-boiled eggs, and low-calorie vegetables on the days when the cafeteria served fried chicken or macaroni and cheese to the other students. He rounded out lunch with whole-wheat bread and skim milk. The Drummonds also enlisted the support of their son's teacher, who encouraged Tommy to make these lower-calorie selections. The teacher was able to smooth the way when other children asked why Tommy got to eat something special.

Housekeepers and Caregivers

With two-career couples becoming the American norm, many families find they must rely on a housekeeper or caregiver to manage their home and their children. If this is the case in your household, it is important to have a discussion with the caregiver about the Stoplight Diet. You might even ask the person to read this book, which makes it more likely that he or she will be able to adhere to the program's principles. You should ask your housekeeper or caregiver to shop only for green and yellow foods, and, most important, to encourage and monitor your children's success with the diet when you cannot be there to do so. Perhaps the caregiver will want to follow the Stoplight Diet too!

On Their Own

There will always be times when your children will have to make decisions for themselves. You cannot be around 100 percent of the time to support their efforts on the Stoplight Diet. But you can lay the groundwork that will influence how your children will eat when you are not present.

· *Teach your children to plan ahead.* You can help your child role-play how he (or she) will behave at a party — how he will control his eating of red foods. We recommend that children eat no more than one red food during celebrations. A few days before the party, children should be especially careful about their calories and should eat no red foods. Help your child to anticipate what may be served at the party. Tell him to look at all the red foods offered and choose the one he wants to eat. Encourage him to ask for a small portion. Be sure to praise your child when he follows through with this plan. If he is unsuccessful, do not get angry. Instead, help him determine how he could have done better. Then encourage him to try again at the next party.

• *Provide low-calorie alternative snacks for your children to have after school.* It is, of course, best not to eat anything after school. But in two-career families, parents often cannot be home after school and may find that their children raid the refrigerator and cupboards in their absence. By not having red foods in the house, you are a step ahead of them. But children can also gain weight by eating too many yellow foods. If your child must snack after school, make sure that there is fruit, juice, or other low-calorie items. One mother we know packed a special after-school snack in a plastic bag and placed it in the refrigerator with a note for her son. Some days she packed celery and carrot sticks along with a small container of apple juice. Other days she left twelve grapes (carefully counted) and two sections of graham cracker. Her son enjoyed the treats and happily recorded them, and she knew that he was not eating more food than he should.

• *Prepare your children for special outings with friends.* Whether they go to the latest movie or attend a ball game, food is bound to be a temptation when your children are with friends. Planning is the key. When possible, pack homemade popcorn for your children and their friends to take to the movies. Commercially prepared corn is usually popped in coconut oil and is very high in saturated fat. If it is not possible to pop your own corn, encourage your children to buy just a small box of popcorn and to order it without butter.

Careful food choices are possible at sporting events as well. One slice of cheese pizza and a diet drink is a fairly low-calorie meal. So is one hot dog with a bun, washed down with a diet drink or juice.

• *Camp can provide a special challenge to children on the Stoplight Diet.* Food at day camp is easier to control than food at overnight camp, where all meals will be prepared by the camp cook. Day camps that require the camper to pack a lunch can easily be adapted to the Stoplight Diet. You and your child can simply choose nonfattening foods for lunch. Overnight camps and day camps that provide lunch may require more work. Consult with your child's counselor and seek help from cooks and camp directors.

Week 7 Quiz

This is our last reading quiz. As before, the questions are designed to make sure you understand what you have read in this chapter and earlier ones. Review any sections that give you difficulty. Remember to pass the quiz on to your spouse and have your children read their corresponding chapter and take the quiz that follows it. Then discuss the chapter and the quiz with them to see if they have any questions.

Answer true or false:

1. To keep from gaining back the pounds you have lost, you and your children need to be in control of your environment.

2. To reduce the temptation to overeat, you should continue to keep all red foods outside the home.

3. It is acceptable to eat dinner while watching television.

4. Eating three meals a day is not important when you are trying to lose weight or maintain weight loss over the long run.

5. Television watching should be limited to three hours a day.

6. It is best to allow your children to watch television only in the afternoon, after they come home from school.

7. When following the Stoplight Diet, you must plan ahead to reduce the chance of backsliding during holidays and other special occasions.

8. *Cue control* is the term psychologists use to describe the conditions that prompt us to feel hungry or sleepy, or make us want to exercise.

Ten-year-old Jim and his father love to watch televised pro football games on Sunday afternoons. While they cheer for their favorite team, they munch on potato chips and drink soda pop.

Now that Jim and his father are on the Stoplight Diet, they realize how many calories they consume each Sunday afternoon during the football season.

9. What cue do Jim and his father respond to when they open the bag of potato chips and drink the soda pop?_____

10. What could Jim and his father do during the games to decrease the number of calories they consume?_____

Nine-year-old Christine is excited because she has been invited to seven Christmas parties this year. But she is also a little worried. She has lost 10 pounds on the Stoplight Diet. But she knows that there will be many temptations at the parties — especially the ones her grandmothers are throwing — and she does not want to gain weight during the Christmas season.

11. What could Christine take to the parties as a treat for her friends?

_____

12. What could Christine's mother say to Christine's grandmothers to make the parties easier for Christine?_____

_____

13. If Christine wants to eat red foods at some of the parties, what should she do?_____

_____

Answers

1. True
2. True
3. False
4. False
5. False (It should be limited to one hour per day.)
6. False (Television is best watched in the evening rather than the afternoon, when children could be outdoors playing.)
7. True
8. True
9. Watching football Sunday afternoons on television.
10. Eat unbuttered popcorn instead of chips, or, better yet, save the money they spend on snacks and use it to go to a sporting event.
11. Low-calorie snacks or party favors that do not involve food.
12. "Christine has been working hard to control her weight. She has worked very hard to lose weight and has done an excellent job. Please continue to help her by not tempting her with high-calorie foods."
13. Preplan what she eats during the week before the party and avoid all red foods so she can have some at the celebrations and still stay within the limit.

Week 8
Following the
Stoplight Signals
Forever

Just seven weeks ago, you decided that you had to help your children lose their excess weight, safely and permanently. In the very first week of the Stoplight Diet program, you began a series of changes that continues to unfold a fuller, healthier world for your entire family.

Today, you know how to lose weight. So do your children. But even better, you are putting that knowledge to work. Your family now shares the success of many other Stoplight Diet families. Your children will never again be the victims of low self-esteem, a poor body image, or the vicious teasing of classmates. They are now in control of what they eat. They know about nutrition and how to exercise. They have learned valuable lessons that will last them a lifetime.

These last seven weeks have been a beginning — a very good beginning. But they are merely the foundation of the new life-style you and your family are building. It is now up to you to continue constructing that life-style. Keep in mind what numerous studies of behavior modification have shown: it takes a minimum of six months before a new behavior becomes an ingrained habit. Your family must remain vigilant to prevent the old ways from slowly creeping back into your daily lives.

By now, your children have lost weight. But they may need to trim additional pounds before they reach the ideal weight for someone their height, age, and sex. (You can recheck their measurements against the norms listed in appendix A.) There is no exact timetable for weight loss. Have your children strictly adhere to the Stoplight Diet and continue to exercise until they drop the remaining pounds. They will gradually lose all the weight necessary during the upcoming weeks or perhaps months.

Once your children reach their goal weight, have them stay within their Stoplight Diet calorie range for at least another week to two weeks. This allows their bodies to overcome temporary fluctuations. Carefully track their weight during this time to make sure that it does not go back higher than the ideal weight.

When you are certain that a child's weight has reached the ideal, you can stabilize it by slowly increasing the number of calories he or she eats. Add 25 to 50 calories a day for younger children — those six to seven years old, who burn fewer calories. Older children may be allowed to eat an additional 100 calories a day, for a revised total calorie limit of 1,300 calories a day.

These additional calories should come from the Basic Four food groups. Continue to avoid junk foods and other red foods. Older children could get these extra calories by drinking an additional glass of milk each day (80 calories) and adding an afternoon snack of half an apple (about 20 calories). Younger children could simply have an extra piece of fruit.

It is particularly important during this period that your children keep weighing themselves every day and that they chart their weight. You then can make sure that they do not start to gain weight. They also must continue to record what they eat and to tally calories each day. If they do gain weight, you need to know exactly how many calories they have been eating in order to cut back accordingly. Explain the process to your children. They need to know that the "extra" calories they eat must be planned carefully and their weight must be checked closely so that it can be stabilized at their goal.

If your older children do not gain weight after eating 1,300 calories a day for one to two weeks, then add another 100 calories a day to their diet. This raises their daily intake to 1,400 calories a day. Follow the same procedure as before. Keep them at 1,400 calories for a week or two and track their weight carefully. If they do not gain weight during one to two weeks at this level, increase their daily calorie intake to 1,500 a day. (For younger children, increase by 25 to 50 calories a day.)

Continue increasing calories at the appropriate level for your child's age until you reach a maximum of 2,000 calories a day for children ten years old and younger. For children aged eleven to seventeen years, the top limit is about 2,800 calories. But remember, never increase calories by more than 100 calories a day for older children; and once you have added these 100 calories, keep your child at that level for a minimum of a week, and preferably for two. It is essential to make this a gradual increase.

If your older child begins to gain weight at a particular calorie level, cut back on intake by 100 calories for a week or so and see if the weight gain stops. If it does not stop, subtract another 100 calories. Keep your child at that level and see if his or her weight stabilizes. If it does not, scale back yet another 100 calories, and so forth, until you determine the correct calorie maintenance level for your child. (For younger children, subtract 25 to 50 calories a day.)

Do not be surprised if your family experiences occasional backslides. They are to be expected. Be sure that you do not take these lapses to mean that you have failed. You have not. The important thing is to weigh yourselves every day. The scale never lies. By keeping a close watch on weight, you and your family will know exactly where you stand. If your children inadvertently gain a pound or so, you can take action right away, rather than wait until they have gained several pounds and weight loss is difficult.

Monitoring your children's weight is extremely important beyond the eight-week period. As they get older, they grow taller, and with that growth come added pounds. Periodically consult appendix A as a guide to whether your children are maintaining body weights that are still within 10 percent of the ideal for them. Every six months, check to see if they need a new goal weight.

Once your children are within their ideal-weight ranges and have maintained those levels for several months, you can start easing off on the requirement that they record their food every day. We do recommend, however, that for one week of every month you have your family record everything they eat, just as they did when they were learning the Stoplight Diet. During this week, everyone should go back to measuring out food or weighing it (if they are no longer doing so).

No family lives in a vacuum. You will continually be enticed by red foods. The rest of the world is not going to give up eating chocolate mousse, fetuccine Alfredo, buttery garlic bread, or any other tantalizing red foods. Neither, perhaps, should your family. But if you want to maintain the weight loss you and your children have worked so hard to achieve — and if you want to continue to eat healthfully — it is essential that you continue to limit the number of red foods consumed each week to four or less. Most important, do not allow red foods back into your house. If a friend or relative brings a red food to your house as a gift, politely taste it and courteously send the rest home with your guest. If that will not work, give the red food away to a neighbor or discreetly throw it out. Do not let the sun set twice while you have a red food in your house — and do not eat a red food unless you are away from home.

Your family represents a new breed of pioneers: people who are changing the way they eat and exercise to ensure better health. A higher-fiber, lower-fat, lower-calorie diet, well-balanced meals, regular physical activity — your children stand to reap many benefits from this superior life-style, including a lower risk of such conditions as heart disease, high blood pressure, cancer, adult-onset diabetes, and, of course, obesity.

Linda Gregg's family of four lost a total of 100 pounds on the Stoplight Diet. "We've overcome thirty years of bad eating habits in two months. We still watch what we eat and we'll never go back to the way we were." Like the Greggs, your family has already begun a new, healthy life-style. Why not make it last forever?

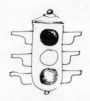

Part Two

THE STOPLIGHT DIET
FOR CHILDREN

What This
Book Is About

Have you ever been teased about your weight? We know many children who have been teased a lot. They've been called names like Tubby and Fatso. They didn't like it very much. In fact, it made them feel hurt and angry. These children told us that they often wished they were not overweight. But they said they did not know how to lose weight.

We are going to show you and your family how to lose weight. We are also going to help you exercise and develop your body to be fit and stronger than it is today. We will do this through the Stoplight Diet.

When someone loses weight by cutting back on what they usually eat, it's known as "going on a diet." Maybe you've tried to diet yourself. The children we talked to found that dieting was not their favorite thing to do. If you have ever tried to diet before, perhaps you've found that it wasn't much fun. We have a friend named Josh who felt the same way. Josh is ten years old, and he's been trying to lose weight since he was eight. Josh is the youngest in his family. He has one brother, whose name is Tim. Tim is fifteen years old and he can be a big tease.

When Josh went on a diet, he tried very hard not to eat fattening foods. He said "No thank you" to french fries. He turned down ice cream. He drank only one Coke instead of three or four. He even tried to give up eating chocolate-chip cookies — his favorite food.

For a day or so, Josh did really well. But then he would see Tim dipping into the ice cream. Or he'd watch Tim pour himself another Coke. The real tough part came when Tim would eat a whole bag of Josh's favorite chocolate-chip cookies. When that happened, Josh found he just couldn't stick to the diet anymore. It was too hard watching Tim and the rest of his family eat all the foods that Josh wanted to eat too.

So Josh stopped his diet and gained weight again. Sometimes Josh had trouble running as fast as his friends. Then his teammates in soccer began making fun of him during games because he couldn't run as fast as they did. Josh quit the team at the end of the season. One day, Josh took a long look at himself in the mirror and was surprised by what he saw. He looked fat. His belly stuck out and his legs looked as if they were twice as big as his older brother's. Josh never told anyone about how bad he felt. He was so embarrassed about his fat legs that he would not wear shorts in the summer — even when the temperature hit 104 degrees.

Josh might have refused to wear shorts for the rest of his life, except that something wonderful and unexpected happened one day. He and his parents were watching television when a commercial flashed on the screen. It said, "Wanted: families with overweight children for a new diet program."

"Honey," Josh's mother said to his father. "Listen to this commercial. Maybe we ought to call and find out about it." Josh's father grabbed a pencil and wrote down the telephone number that appeared on the television screen. His mother called the next day, and a week after that, Josh and his parents were on their way to starting the Stoplight Diet with a large group of other children and their families at the University of Pittsburgh.

Josh was a little worried. He wondered if going to the University of Pittsburgh would be like going to see the doctor. (It turned out that it wasn't.) Josh met a lot of nice people, who weighed him and measured how tall he was.

They also determined how much fat Josh had on his body. It was all very painless.

Josh and his parents waited a little while. Then they went into an office where a woman told them that they could join the Stoplight Diet program. She explained that Josh and his family should come back next week for another visit. She told Josh that he would meet other children who would also be starting the Stoplight Diet program. She said that the program would help him lose weight. Josh liked hearing that, but wondered if this diet would really work.

Then the woman told him the best news. She said that everyone in his family — his mother, his father, even Tim — would be starting the Stoplight Diet too.

"Even Tim!" Josh exclaimed. "I think I'm going to like this diet."

And he did. Over the next several months, Josh worked very hard and learned a lot. He learned about eating foods that are good for him. He learned about exercise. He learned about weighing himself every day on the bathroom scale. But most of all, Josh learned how to lose weight.

Josh lost a total of 11 pounds over five months. He found he could run a lot faster. He even started taking karate. Other people stopped teasing him about his weight. He still grew out of his clothes — not because they became too tight, but because they became too loose! Josh changed a lot. He's very proud of what he's done.

You can do what Josh did. By reading this book with your mom and dad, you are going to learn everything that Josh and his parents learned. These lessons are going to teach you how to lose weight, and keep it off forever.

Why do we call our diet program the Stoplight Diet? It's named after the signals on a traffic light. Most traffic lights have three signals. You know that the green signal means "Go." The yellow signal tells you "Caution" or "Be careful," because the light is about to change. The red signal, of course, means "Stop!"

We have placed all the food that you eat into three different groups. These are called *red foods, yellow foods,* and *green foods.* By thinking about the three different signals on a stoplight every time you eat, you can make good decisions about which foods to eat.

But you should also know that a food's real color does not always match its food group color. For instance, when Josh first started the Stoplight Diet, he thought that a red apple would be a red food. But he learned that all apples are in the group of yellow foods since they are not very fattening. Josh also thought that an avocado would be a green food. But since avocados have a lot of fat, they are grouped with the red foods.

You will soon find that the real color of most foods is not important on the Stoplight Diet. What matters is the color of the food group. Like Josh, you will learn which foods belong to which color groups.

Red foods on the Stoplight Diet are very fattening. That means that they make people gain weight. When you think of eating a red food, remember the red light on a traffic signal and *stop*.

Yellow foods on our diet are less fattening than red foods. In fact, most foods that we eat fall into the yellow food group. What does a yellow signal tell you? "Caution," or "Be careful" — and that is what you need to do when you eat yellow foods.

Green foods on the Stoplight Diet are not fattening. Like the green signal on a traffic light, these foods mean "Go." It's okay to eat green foods, almost as many as you want.

Josh and his family aren't the only ones who went on the Stoplight Diet. We know children from more than 250 families who have already lost weight on the Stoplight Diet. And the Stoplight Diet will help you lose weight too!

Each week, you and your family will read a chapter from this book. By reading these chapters and doing what they teach you, you can lose weight and feel great about yourself.

At the end of each week's chapter you will find a quiz to take. Unlike the quizzes that your teachers give you in school, these won't be graded, and the answers are included in the book. (But no fair peeking at the answers until you have finished the quiz!)

When you are done reading the chapter and have tried

the quiz, show your answers to your mom and dad. They will talk to you about what you have read. They can also answer any questions that you may have about the Stoplight Diet. We want you to understand as much as you can about our diet program. The more you understand, the easier it will be to lose weight.

Even if you don't need to lose weight, you can get something out of this book. It will help you learn about eating right and exercising so that you will never get fat and will have a long and healthy life. It will also give you the facts you need to help someone else who may be trying to lose weight. Just as Josh's older brother, Tim, learned how to help him lose weight, you can help make the Stoplight Diet a success for your brother or sister.

But the best part of the Stoplight Diet is this: It will teach you how to change your life forever. We will show you how to lose weight and teach you how to keep it off for good.

Like Josh, you will find that you need never be teased about your weight again.

Week 1
Learn the
Stoplight Signals

Red, Yellow, or Green?

This week, we are going to teach you about the signals on the Stoplight Diet. You already know a lot about these signals because they are patterned after the red, yellow, and green signals on a traffic light.

We designed the diet this way to make it easier for you to remember which foods will help you lose weight and which foods will make you fat.

The good foods — the ones that will help you lose weight — are *green foods* and *yellow foods*. Just like the green signal on the traffic light, foods in the green group tell you "Go." You can eat almost as many of these foods as you like.

Yellow foods are also good foods, but they must be eaten with a little more caution — just the way the yellow signal on a traffic light cautions you to be careful because the signal is about to change to red. If you eat too many yellow foods, you will not lose weight. They can even make you gain weight if you are not careful.

Red foods are very fattening. They make people gain weight — something we know you do not want to do. When you see a red food, think of the red light on a traffic signal and STOP. On the Stoplight Diet, you will eat only four red foods or fewer each week.

Food Is the Body's Fuel

Have you ever wondered why some people are fat, some people are thin, and some people are somewhere in between? Many scientists have asked that same question.

They have learned that our bodies are like engines. In order to run, they need fuel. The fuel our bodies burn is food. Food allows our lungs to work so that we can breathe. It keeps our hearts beating, and our brains working so that we can think and talk and move.

Food also gives our muscles strength. We can hit a home run, or ride a bicycle, or jump rope because food provides the energy.

Sometimes, though, our bodies get too much food. The body does not want to waste this food so it stores it. The place our bodies store this extra fuel is called fat.

Everyone's body has some fat on it. Even your skinniest friend has fat. And it makes sense for the body to store a little fat. If something suddenly happened so that your body could not get any food, your fat would help out. Your body could burn your fat as fuel until you could get food again.

The trouble comes when you feed your body much more food than it can burn off through exercise. It keeps storing more and more fat. Your weight keeps going higher and higher. Being too heavy can hurt your health and make you feel bad about yourself. That's what happened to our friend Josh when he became fat.

The Stoplight Diet will help you lose weight. To keep your body from storing extra fat, you must give it smaller amounts of food, or fuel. How can you tell how much food you are eating? In two ways. The first is by counting *calories*.

Calories measure how much fuel is in food. For instance, one slice of bread has 80 calories. A glass of skim milk has 80 calories too. A hamburger patty has much more fuel, about 220 calories. You get the idea. (In the back of this book, on pages 194 to 221, we tell you the number of calories in all kinds of foods.)

The second way to tell how much food you eat is by measuring the size of each serving. Your parents keep special tools for this purpose in your kitchen. Measuring cups and measuring spoons are one kind of tool used to keep track of the amount of food in each portion. Your parents may also have a scale to weigh food. It is very important for you and your family to use these tools to tell exactly how much food you are eating at each meal. If you have any questions about using measuring cups or spoons, ask your mom and dad. They will show you how to use them.

Check It Out: "The Stoplight Diet Food Guide"

Besides measuring food and counting calories, you and your family will keep track of the various *types* of foods that you eat. One way you will do this is by counting the number of "red," "yellow," or "green" foods you eat each day.

No one is born knowing whether a food is in the red food group, the yellow food group, or the green one. This is something that everyone must learn — even your mom and dad. To help you learn, we have written "The Stoplight Diet Food Guide." Some children who have used it have nicknamed it "the red, yellow, green guide." You can find this guide in the back of this book, starting on page 194.

Every time you eat a food, look it up in "the red, yellow, green guide." The guide will tell you which group the food is in, and your parents can help if you're not sure. Pretty soon, even without checking, you will know yourself which foods are "red," which foods are "yellow," and which foods are "green."

The food guide tells you something else that is very important: the number of calories that are in the food you eat. As you now know, calories are a way of measuring how much fuel is in what you eat. To lose weight on the Stoplight Diet, you will need to eat only a certain number of calories each day.

If you are eight to twelve years old, you need to eat between 900 to 1,200 total calories each day. If you are six or seven years old, you need to eat 1,000 to 1,200 calories each day. By eating this number of calories daily, you will lose about ½ pound to 1 pound a week — or even more if you exercise more often.

Your Stoplight Diet Habit Book

To keep track of the calories you eat, your mom and dad are going to help you fill out a daily food chart and make what we call a Stoplight Diet habit book. Everyone in your family will have one. You may want to draw or color a special picture or design for the cover of yours.

The habit book is like a diary. It is where you will write down all the food that you eat each day. The best way to do this is by listing what you have eaten as soon as you're done eating it. That way you won't forget anything. What if you don't have your habit book with you? You can write yourself a note and then add the foods to your book as soon as you can.

Remember to write down anything and everything you eat or drink. That includes the catsup you put on your hamburger at lunch or the snack you have at your friend's house. All this food needs to be listed in your habit book.

This week, your parents will start to teach you how to write down your food. By looking ahead to page 137, you can see how Josh listed what he ate one day. As you can tell, there are several other things that you will learn how to note in your habit book. One is the number of "green foods," "yellow foods," and "red foods" that you eat.

Red Food Alert

As you now know, foods in the red food group are very fattening. But what exactly does that mean? It means that red foods contain a lot of calories. By eating red foods you give your body too much fuel. Remember that when your body gets too much fuel, it stores more fat. If your body stores more fat, you will not be able to lose weight. So on the Stoplight Diet, you and your family will eat only four red foods or fewer each week. The fewer you eat, the more weight you will lose.

How can you tell if a food is red? The best way is to check "The Stoplight Diet Food Guide" in the back of this book. Another way is to remember that foods that are very sweet-tasting are often red foods. The sweet taste usually means that a food has lots of sugar in it. Soda pop is one example of a red food that is sweet. Candy is another example.

Many red foods are also very high in *fat*. The fat in your food contains many calories. And the more calories you eat, the more likely you are to put on weight. Eating lots of fat also makes it much harder for you to lose weight.

Figuring out which foods are high in fat is a very hard thing to do just by taste. Butter and margarine have a lot of fat, so they are red foods. So is ice cream. Whole milk also has a lot of fat. But skim milk has almost none and counts as a yellow food.

Deep-fried foods are almost always red foods. For example, fried chicken, fried shrimp, french fries, potato chips, and corn chips are red foods. But you will be happy to know that pretzels and popcorn — served without butter — count as yellow foods.

The more you know about red foods the better. This week, your parents may ask for your help in throwing out all the red foods in your house. Your mom and dad have agreed not to buy any more red foods. From now on, you and your family will not eat red foods at home, but you may eat four red foods (or fewer) a week at someone else's house, at school, or at a restaurant.

Each time you eat a red food, it is important to write it down in your habit book. You also need to record where you ate it and put a star by this food to show you ate it away from home. Your parents will show you how. Remember: eat no more than four red foods a week.

Weighing In

Every day, our friend Josh does something that you will do too. Josh weighs himself on the bathroom scale. When Josh first started the Stoplight Diet, all the members of his family weighed themselves. Josh's mom and dad also checked to see how tall he was. Then they made a chart like the one on the next page for every member of the family.

Josh and his family use these charts to track how much weight they lose. Your parents will do this for you too. They will also help you figure out how much weight to lose — that is, they will help you set a *goal weight.*

You will weigh yourself each day, just like Josh does. It is best if you weigh yourself at the same time every day and either weigh yourself without clothes on or while wearing just underwear. Josh weighs himself in the morning before he eats breakfast. Then he writes down his weight on the chart his mom and dad gave him. By connecting the dots on the graph, Josh and his parents can tell if his weight is going down, staying the same, or going up. You will get to do this too.

You can see from Josh's graph that on Monday he weighed 111 pounds. On Tuesday, his weight stayed the same, 111 pounds. And on Wednesday, he still weighed 111 pounds. (At least he wasn't gaining weight!) By Thursday, Josh had lost 1 pound; he weighed 110. His weight stayed at 110 pounds on Friday, Saturday, and Sunday.

You have learned a lot about eating this week. Let's go over some of the things you will want to remember:

· Eating green and yellow foods helps you lose weight.
· Write down everything that you eat each day in your Stoplight Diet habit book.
· Look in "The Stoplight Diet Food Guide" to see what type of food — red, yellow, or green — you are about to eat.
· If you are not sure about whether a food is red, yellow, or green, ask your mom or dad before eating it.
· Weigh yourself every day and mark your weight on your chart.
· Help your parents throw out all the red foods in your house.
· Eat no more than four red foods each week. Try your best not to eat any at all. You will lose weight faster.

Name ___Josh___ Week Number _1_

Goal Weight _100_

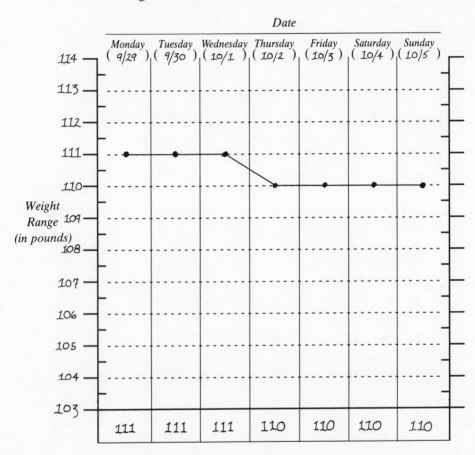

Date

Josh's Daily Weight Chart

Now that you have read about the Stoplight Diet signals, try our quiz. Be sure to show your answers to your mom and dad when you are finished. They will answer any questions you may have.

Week 1 Quiz

Answer true or false to the following questions:

1. Everyone in your family can go on the Stoplight Diet with you, even if they don't all need to lose weight.   True   False

2. The Stoplight Diet will help you lose weight.   True   False

3. Red foods are very high in calories.   True   False

4. Green foods are very low in calories.   True   False

5. When you eat yellow foods, you have to use caution.   True   False

6. Most foods that are fried are low in calories and will help you lose weight.   True   False

7. To lose weight, you must decrease the number of calories you eat.   True   False

8. You need to weigh yourself every day on the Stoplight Diet.   True   False

9. You may eat ten red foods a week on the Stoplight Diet.   True   False

10. It is okay to have a few red foods in your house.   True   False

Use "The Stoplight Diet Food Guide" — "the red, yellow, green guide" on pages 194 to 221 — to find the color group for each of these foods.

Food	*Color*
11. Apple	_____
12. Whole milk	_____
13. Popcorn (air-popped)	_____
14. Turkey (no skin)	_____
15. Baked chicken (no skin)	_____

Food	Color
16. Fried chicken	_____
17. Candy bar	_____
18. Grapes	_____
19. Pretzels	_____
20. Shredded wheat	_____
21. Peas	_____

Use the food guide to figure out the number of calories in each of the foods below. Then show whether each food is red, yellow, or green.

	Calories	Color
22. 8 ounces of Coke	_____	_____
23. 8 ounces of Diet Coke	_____	_____
24. ⅓ cup of apple juice	_____	_____
25. 1 cup of popcorn (air-popped)	_____	_____
26. 1 small baked potato	_____	_____
27. ½ cup of rice	_____	_____
28. ½ cup of plain spaghetti	_____	_____
29. 1 cup of celery	_____	_____
30. ½ cup of carrots	_____	_____

Answers

1. True	11. yellow	21. yellow
2. True	12. red	22. 95/red
3. True	13. yellow	23. 0/green
4. True	14. yellow	24. 40/yellow
5. True	15. yellow	25. 20/yellow
6. False	16. red	26. 80/yellow
7. True	17. red	27. 80/yellow
8. True	18. yellow	28. 80/yellow
9. False	19. yellow	29. 20/green
10. False	20. yellow	30. 20/green

Week 2
The ABCs of
Smart Eating

Welcome to the second week of the Stoplight Diet.
Are you surprised at how easy it is to write down what you eat and to weigh yourself every day? Our friend Josh was pleased that he now liked getting on the scale every day. Before he went on the Stoplight Diet, Josh used to dread weighing himself. Each time he got on the scale, he weighed more! Josh hated that. It made him feel very bad.

What surprised Josh about the Stoplight Diet is that he began to like weighing himself because the scale reading no longer went up. For a while, it stayed the same. And then, even better, it started to go down. Josh began to lose weight. That made him feel very good. Josh also liked using his diary to record what he ate each day. He realized that writing down what he ate helped him keep track of his calories. By keeping track of his calories — and staying under 1,200 calories a day — Josh began to lose weight.

So did another one of our friends named Kate. Kate and Josh met at the Stoplight Diet program, run by the University of Pittsburgh. Kate is also ten years old.

Like Josh, Kate lost a lot of weight on the Stoplight Diet. In fact, she lost a total of 25 pounds in six months.

If you met Kate today, you would never guess that she

was once fat. Kate likes that. She is very proud of how she looks now.

Being slim is a big change for Kate. She used to hate to look in the mirror. Now she loves to admire herself. It reminds her of what a good job she has done in losing weight.

There is another change for Kate too. "I have a lot of friends now," Kate says. Before, when she was fat, many of Kate's classmates made fun of her. That made Kate feel very bad. She became shy, and sometimes would not talk.

But now, Kate smiles often. She also talks a lot. Sometimes her older sister, Jenny, even thinks that Kate talks *too* much.

Josh and Kate did not become slim by magic. They worked very hard to lose weight. They paid attention to the red, yellow, and green foods. They carefully counted calories. They wrote down everything that they ate. If they snacked, they ate green or yellow foods like carrot and celery sticks. Sometimes they saved an apple from their lunch for an afternoon snack. Other times, they drank a small glass of orange juice when they came home from school.

Now that they have lost weight, Josh and Kate are working just as hard to make sure that they never get fat again. The way they stay slim is by remembering some important lessons about good food habits. We call them the ABCs of smart eating.

· *Lesson A: Eat balanced meals from the Basic Four food groups.* Last week we learned about red, yellow, and green foods. Now we'll take it one step further. Most of the food we eat falls into one of four main groups. These Basic Four food groups are:

> Protein
> Grains
> Fruits and Vegetables
> Dairy

To stay healthy, it is important to eat balanced meals. Balanced meals contain foods from all or most of these food groups.

For example, Josh loves to eat cereal for breakfast. He always puts fruit on top of the cereal. Strawberries are his favorite fruit, but he also likes blueberries and peaches. Once Josh has the cereal and the fruit in a bowl, he pours skim milk on top and then he gets himself a glass of orange juice.

Josh really likes this breakfast. It tastes good and he knows it is good for him. Josh is also very smart in choosing his breakfast. His cereal is a food from the *grain* group. The strawberries and the orange juice are both members of the *fruits-and-vegetables* group. And the skim milk Josh pours over his cereal is part of the *dairy* group. Sometimes Josh also eats a soft-boiled egg, which is part of the *protein* group.

You can see that Josh picks his breakfast very wisely. By choosing foods from three of the Basic Four groups, he eats a balanced meal and shows how much he has learned about nutrition.

Nutrition is the study of what people eat and how the body uses food. Like Josh, you have already learned a lot about nutrition.

You know, for example, that most of what you eat comes from the four main types of food. These are the protein group, the grains group, the fruits-and-vegetables group, and the dairy group.

Protein foods are important because they give you energy. In fact, your body must have them in order to grow. Many foods with lots of protein in them also contain other things your body needs. *Iron,* a type of *mineral,* is one example. Your blood uses the iron to keep you healthy.

Vitamins are another example. Your body cannot live without vitamins. One important type of vitamin you get from protein foods is called *niacin.* Niacin is needed by your brain and helps other parts of your body.

What foods have a lot of protein? Red meat, chicken, and turkey are high in protein. So are fish, eggs, and nuts.

Many people think that eating a lot of protein is very healthful. It usually is. But if you eat too much protein, your body will store it as fat. So be careful not to overdo the protein.

Protein foods count as yellow foods on the Stoplight Diet unless they contain a lot of fat or calories. Then they are red foods. Here is one example: Fried chicken is a red food. But baked or broiled chicken without the skin has less fat and is a yellow food.

Grains, the second food group, are usually very good to eat too. Like protein foods, they give you lots of energy. There are many members of the grains group. Bread is one of the best-known grain foods. The cereal that you eat at breakfast is another grain. Other members of the grains group are bagels, crackers, spaghetti, noodles, rolls, and rice.

When you eat foods from the grain group, your body gets iron, which is important for your blood. It also gets some "B vitamins." As we said earlier, your body needs vitamins to live. And guess what? Grains have some protein in them too.

Most foods in the grain group are low in calories. On the Stoplight Diet, they are usually yellow foods. But if you put a lot of fattening butter or margarine on them, they count as red foods. Here's why: If you butter a piece of bread, you add fat to it. If you put a creamy sauce on your noodles, you add fat and many calories. Adding honey, sugar, jelly, jam, or syrup also can turn yellow grain foods into red foods. It's smart to eat yellow foods plain, so that they stay low in calories.

Fruits and vegetables, the third food group, are very good to eat. They are low in calories and they taste delicious. Almost all fruits and vegetables count as green or as yellow foods.

When you eat fruits and vegetables your body gets lots of vitamins, especially vitamin A and vitamin C. Vitamins, as you know, are very good for your health. Some scientists can even show that people who eat many fruits and vegetables are less likely to get diseases such as cancer.

Dairy foods are the fourth basic food group. The best-known dairy foods are milk, cheese, and yogurt.

Dairy foods are very good foods to eat and drink because

they give your body *calcium*. Calcium, like iron, is a mineral. It helps your bones grow and keeps them strong.

Dairy products have another mineral called *phosphorus,* which is very good for your bones too. When you eat or drink dairy foods, your body also gets a lot of protein, plus vitamin D.

But unless you choose your dairy foods carefully, you can also get a lot of fat from them. For instance, whole milk is a red food, but skim milk — which has the fat taken out of it, or "skimmed off" — is very low in fat. Skim milk is a yellow food. It is much better to drink skim milk. Josh's family used to drink only whole milk. That is one reason why they needed to lose weight.

Because it contains a lot of fat, an 8-ounce glass of whole milk has 160 calories. But skim milk contains almost no fat and has only 80 calories per 8-ounce glass. By switching from whole milk to skim milk, Josh and his family saved 80 calories a glass. That's a lot of calories!

Many cheeses and yogurt made with whole milk are also very high in fat. Always check with your mom or dad before eating these foods.

· *Lesson B: Make sure that you eat enough servings from each of the Basic Four food groups.* Here is what to eat every day:

It is best to eat *two servings of protein foods every day,* for a total of 4 ounces. You can use a kitchen scale to measure how many ounces of protein foods you eat. Our friend Josh often eats a turkey sandwich for lunch. Then he has a small piece of chicken as his protein for dinner. The total of the protein foods he eats is just 4 ounces from these two meals.

Kate is also careful about how many protein foods she eats. Some days Kate eats a cheese sandwich for lunch. One slice of American cheese weighs about 1 ounce. Then Kate's dad fixes shrimp — one of Kate's favorite foods — for dinner. If Kate eats one slice of cheese in her sandwich at lunch, she can have 3 ounces of shrimp at dinner — for a total of 4 ounces.

You need to eat *four servings of grains every day*. Here is what Josh does: He eats cereal for breakfast. Then he has a sandwich made with two slices of bread for lunch, and he eats some rice at dinner. Sometimes instead of the rice he will have spaghetti. Other nights, his parents serve macaroni. If you have questions about which foods are in the grains group, ask your mom or dad for help.

You need to eat *at least four servings of fruits and vegetables every day*. This is what Kate does: She drinks a small glass of orange juice at breakfast. (Orange juice, grapefruit juice, tangerines, lemons, and limes all have a lot of vitamin C.) At lunch, Kate eats celery and carrot sticks. (Carrots have a lot of vitamin A.) Kate's mom also puts lettuce and a slice of tomato on Kate's sandwich. (Tomatoes have a lot of vitamin C.) Kate usually has a piece of fruit with lunch. Her favorite is a peach. Then, at dinner, Kate's dad likes to cook broccoli. (Broccoli has a lot of vitamin A.) Sometimes, Kate's parents cook peas, another good vegetable. They also like to eat corn and often start dinner with a salad.

For dessert, Kate likes to have a small bowl of berries. Strawberries and blueberries are her first choices. During the winter, Kate's parents buy unsweetened, frozen berries. Kate lets them thaw for a few minutes before eating them. Sometimes, Kate's mom puts a banana in the freezer. It tastes quite good.

Finally, you need to eat or drink *three servings of dairy foods every day*. Josh does this by drinking skim milk with each meal. Kate likes cottage cheese as one of her daily servings. Ask your mom or dad to help you pick out dairy foods and to check whether you are eating three balanced meals each day.

· *Lesson C: Eat no more than four red foods a week.* You already know this rule and why it's important: red foods are very fattening. If you can eat fewer than four red foods, you will lose weight faster and you will eat more healthfully.

Eating foods that have too much fat means that it will be hard for you to lose weight. Also, too much fat in your food is not good for your body. You probably know that your heart pumps blood all through your body, from your head to your toes. The blood travels through many small, soft tubes that are connected to your heart. These tubes are called *blood vessels,* and there are two main types: *arteries* and *veins.* (If you look at the underside of your wrist, you can see parts of these blood vessels. Do you see bluish lines? They are veins.)

Scientists now know that if you eat too much fat, your arteries can become clogged as you grow older. You don't have to be very old to have clogged blood vessels. Some people in their twenties already have this problem. When the vessels of the heart become clogged, or stuffed up, a heart attack can happen. That is very dangerous and some-times deadly.

But scientists also know how to help prevent our vessels from getting clogged. They suggest that we all eat much less fat. This is another reason why it is important to eat few red foods.

Josh and Kate now do this. But it was not always easy for them. Kate remembers one really hot summer day when an ice-cream truck drove through her neighborhood ringing its bell.

Kate was outside playing with her friend Julie. As soon as the truck stopped, it seemed as if everybody in the neigh-borhood lined up to buy ice cream.

Julie's mother gave Julie money to buy an ice-cream bar for Julie and for Kate. But Kate had to say "No thank you" to Julie because ice cream is a red food.

Kate felt the tears well up in her eyes as she watched everyone else get ice cream. Just when she thought she could not keep from crying, Kate heard her mom call.

"Kate, come here, I've got something for you," her mom said. Kate's mother stood at the front door. She had some-thing in her hand and she was smiling.

Kate ran to see her mother. "Mom, I said 'No thank you' to ice cream, but it's really hot today," Kate said. "I really wish I could have some."

"I know you do, honey," Kate's mom said. "I'm really proud of you for turning down the ice cream. But I've got a surprise for you. I froze some fruit juice on a stick in the freezer. It's nice and cold. It tastes really good, and it's not a red food. You can give one to Julie too if you want."

Kate dried her eyes. She and her mom hugged each other. "Thanks a lot, Mom," Kate said. "Now I won't have to write down a red food in my Stoplight Diet diary."

· *Lesson D: Always write down everything that you eat in your Stoplight Diet habit book.* This is another lesson you already know about. Kate's mom helped her remember some foods at first. For instance, sometimes Kate forgot that she had eaten catsup on her hamburger. She sometimes also forgot that she put salad dressing on her lettuce. Kate's mom reminded Kate about eating those foods. Soon, Kate remembered on her own. You will too.

As you know, it is best to write down your food right after eating. When Josh finishes breakfast, he gets out his Stoplight Diet habit book and turns to a daily food chart. First, he writes the day of the week and the date. Then he puts down the time he ate breakfast. Next, he fills in what he ate. He also notes *how much* he ate. Then he checks the food guide at the back of this book and writes down the number of calories for each food. He also shows whether each food is a green or a yellow one. Finally, Josh puts a checkmark to keep track of how many servings from each Basic Four food group he ate.

The chart shown here let's you see how this works. At seven-thirty on Monday morning, September 29, Josh ate two-thirds of a cup of Bran Chex for breakfast. Look at the daily food chart and you will see where he wrote down the cereal. Then he filled in the number of calories, which was 90. Next, he put a "Y" for food color, since the cereal was a yellow food. Finally, he checked the "G" column. This is because the cereal was a member of the grains group.

Josh did the same thing to record the strawberries he ate. He measured the strawberries, so he knew that he ate three-fourths of a cup. Then he looked up "Strawberries" in the food guide (page 205) and wrote down 40 calories. Next, he recorded a "Y" in the food color column. Finally, he

Name ___Josh___   Date ___Monday, Sept. 29___

Time	Food or Drink	Amount	Number of Calories	Food Group Color	Basic Four Food Group P	G	F&V	D
7:30am	Bran Chex	2/3 Cup	90	y		✓		
	Strawberries - plain	3/4 Cup	40	y			✓	
	Orange Juice	1/2 Cup	40	y			✓	
	Skim milk	1 Cup	80	y				✓
12:30pm	Whole-wheat bread	2 slices	160	y		✓✓		
	Turkey	1 ounce	50	y	✓			
	Celery & carrot sticks	1/2 Cup	20	G			✓	
	Apple (small)	1	40	y			✓	
	skim milk	1 Cup	80	y				✓
	Totals							
	Goals		900-1200		2	4	4	3

Josh's Daily Food Chart

placed a checkmark in the "F&V" column. "F&V" stands for fruits and vegetables.

You can see that Josh also remembered to record his glass of orange juice. He also wrote down the skim milk he poured over his cereal. In recording the milk, Josh noted that he used 1 cup. He wrote in 80 for the number of calories. Then he placed a "Y" in the color column. Finally, Josh checked off the "D" column, which stands for "Dairy."

Josh eats lunch at school, and he usually writes down his food as soon as he gets home in the afternoon. For lunch on this day, Josh ate a turkey sandwich on whole-wheat bread and had carrot and celery sticks. He drank a carton of skim milk and then he had an apple for dessert.

Here's how he recorded his food:

Josh first wrote down the time he ate lunch. It was 12:30 P.M. He ate two slices of whole-wheat bread. By looking in "the red, yellow, green guide" he found that two slices add up to 160 calories (80 calories each). He wrote a "Y" in the food color column and then he placed two checkmarks in the "G" column, since each slice counts as one serving from the grains group.

Next, Josh recorded the turkey that he ate on his sandwich. Josh's mother packs his lunch. She told him that she gave him 1 ounce of turkey meat. Josh wrote that down in the "Amount" column. Then he read in the food guide that 3 ounces of turkey meat is 150 calories. Since he ate only 1 ounce, he divided 150 by 3 and wrote in the answer: 50 calories. Turkey is a yellow food, so Josh wrote a "Y" in the food color column. Next, he checked off the "P" column, because turkey is a protein food.

Josh also recorded his celery and carrot sticks — green foods (G) — and the apple that he ate. He marked those fruits and vegetables in the "F&V" column. Finally, Josh looked over what he had recorded and remembered to add the skim milk.

When he is finished eating dinner, Josh will again record what he eats. Then he and his mom or dad will compare their food charts for the day. They will add up all their calories. Josh's parents will also help him check to make sure that he ate enough servings from all the Basic Four food groups. Finally, they will check to see if he ate any red foods. (Josh didn't.)

You and your family will use your Stoplight Diet habit books the same way Josh and his parents did.

· *Lesson E: Stay within the Stoplight Diet calorie range.* When some people go on a diet, they cut back too much on what they eat. Other people skip meals. These are very bad ideas.

People who do diet this way can lose weight. But they usually gain the weight back, because they have not learned how to change what they eat. They don't know about red, yellow, and green foods. They also don't know how to exercise, which helps them keep the pounds off. When they gain the weight back, they feel very discouraged.

You need energy each day. On the Stoplight Diet, you will eat enough fuel to give you plenty of energy. You will also be able to lose weight. If you are at least eight years old, your calorie range is 900 to 1,200 calories. That means you should never eat less than 900 calories or more than 1,200 calories each day. If you are six or seven years old, your Stoplight Diet range is 1,000 to 1,200 calories. Until you turn eight, you should never eat less than 1,000 calories a day or more than 1,200 calories a day.

Now you know the ABCs of smart eating on the Stoplight Diet. Here is the weekly quiz. Remember to ask your mom and dad to look at it with you. If you have any questions, be sure to get their help.

Week 2 Quiz

Answer true or false:

1. Drinking skim milk is good for you.　　True　False
2. Fruits and vegetables have lots of vitamins.　　True　False
3. Chicken, turkey, and hamburger are in the grains food group.　　True　False

4. Meat and fish are in the protein group.	True False
5. It is important to eat balanced meals.	True False
6. Milk, cheese, and yogurt are members of the dairy food group.	True False
7. Dairy foods are very good for your bones.	True False
8. Bread, spaghetti, rice, cereal, and crackers are members of the grain group.	True False
9. You can eat more than four red foods a week on the Stoplight Diet.	True False
10. Most members of the grains group are pretty low in calories and are yellow foods.	True False

Use the food guide in the back of this book to answer which of the Basic Four food groups the foods below belong in. Then show what color they are on the Stoplight Diet. When you write down your answers, use the same initials you would use to record foods in your daily record.

Food	Basic Four Food Group	Color
11. Apple	_____	_____
12. Turkey	_____	_____
13. Rice	_____	_____
14. Carrots	_____	_____
15. Corn	_____	_____
16. Peas	_____	_____
17. Orange juice	_____	_____
18. Shrimp	_____	_____
19. Hamburger	_____	_____
20. Cottage cheese	_____	_____

21. Suppose that you eat a tuna sandwich with lettuce and tomato for lunch. You also have an apple.

    a. The bread you eat in your sandwich is from which Basic Four food group? _____

    b. The tuna is a member of which Basic Four food group? _____

    c. The lettuce and tomato belong to which Basic Four food group? _____

    d. The apple is from which Basic Four food group? _____

    e. What Basic Four food group did you not eat from at lunch? _____

Answers

1. True	10. True	18. P/Y
2. True	11. F&V/Y	19. P/Y
3. False	12. P/Y	20. D/Y
4. True	13. G/Y	21. a. G
5. True	14. F&V/G	b. P
6. True	15. F&V/Y	c. F&V
7. True	16. F&V/Y	d. F&V
8. True	17. F&V/Y	e. D
9. False		

Week 3
Praise and
Privileges

Welcome to the third week of the Stoplight Diet. If you have followed all the instructions so far, then you and your family have been really doing a good job. You probably can even tell a difference in how you feel.

You are also learning a lot. Let's review a few things you have learned during the past two weeks. You have learned about red, yellow, and green foods. You know that food is the body's fuel, and you know why everyone must eat a balanced diet. You have learned about counting calories. You also know now how important it is to weigh yourself every day.

Is your weight starting to go down? If not, don't worry. It will soon. Sometimes it takes a little while for weight loss to begin. The Stoplight Diet is planned so that you will lose weight slowly.

When you lose weight slowly, you learn to change how you eat. This means that the weight you lose will be less likely to come back. We want to make sure that you keep off the pounds that you lose. We know that you want that too.

The important thing is to keep doing everything that you learned so far.

· Weigh yourself every day. Mark your weight on the chart your parents gave you.

· Eat no more than four red foods a week, and never eat them at home.

· Stay within your calorie range. Eat 1,200 calories or less. But remember, always eat at least 900 calories — unless you are younger than eight years old. Then you need to eat at least 1,000 calories a day.

· Ask your parents before eating any food, especially between meals.

· Write down everything that you eat. Try to do this as soon after a meal as possible.

By now, you and your family have thrown out all the red foods in your house. Maybe you miss having them around. That's okay. For the first several weeks, our friend Josh missed red foods too.

Josh kept going into the kitchen to get one of his favorite chocolate-chip cookies. Every time he looked in the cupboard where they were usually kept, they were gone. Then Josh remembered.

"No more red foods in the house," Josh said to himself.

It took a little getting used to. But now, Josh likes having no red foods in his house. He knows that it means he will have fewer chances to gain back the weight he lost.

Praise

Josh is very proud of his body today. He likes the way he looks. Lots of other people — his parents, his older brother, his friends — tell him that they like the way he looks too.

His mother says: "You sure look great, Josh. I'm really impressed with the way you've worked so hard to lose weight."

His father says: "Your hard work really paid off. You are one handsome boy. Look how long and thin your legs are now."

When Josh's parents and friends tell him how good he looks, they are giving him *praise*. Giving praise means telling or showing someone that he or she did a good job. If you do well on a test in school, your parents are very pleased. They tell you how proud they are of you. Their praise makes you feel good.

Everyone likes to be praised. It's also important to know that praise works two ways. This means that the people who *give* the praise feel as good as the people who *get* the praise. One of the lessons we will teach you this week is how to give praise to your parents.

What does praise have to do with losing weight? When you eat no more than 1,200 calories each day for a week, your parents are going to praise you. For instance, your mother might say, "You have done a great job sticking to the calorie limit this week. I am really happy to see how well you've done."

When you write down everything you eat — and especially when you remember to do it yourself, without being reminded — your dad might say to you, "I am really proud of the way you wrote down your food this week without being asked. You seem to really understand how the Stoplight Diet works. That makes me very pleased." Then he might give you a big hug. Praise is going to make you feel very good.

You can help your parents feel good too. When they cook good-tasting, nonfattening green and yellow foods, give them some praise. You might say, "That was a really good meal, Mom." Or you might tell your dad: "That tasted super — and it wasn't fattening either. Thanks."

Look for other reasons to praise your parents too. Like you, your mom and dad are trying to eat better by following the Stoplight Diet. Maybe they are also trying to lose weight. Your praise will help them do so.

When should you praise your mom and dad? Here are some examples:

• Praise them when they do not buy red foods at the store. Josh once told his mother: "Mom, thanks for not buying chocolate-chip cookies for me. I know I asked for them at

the store. But I'm really glad that you didn't buy them. Thanks for being strong and helping me."
· Praise them when they help you review each Stoplight Diet chapter and look over your quiz. You might say, "Thanks, Dad, for taking the time to read this week's chapter with me."
· Praise your mom and dad when they do not eat red foods. Josh told his mother: "Thanks for turning down the potato chips at the party, Mom. Watching you say 'No thank you' helped me not eat potato chips too."
· Praise your parents when they praise you for losing weight. You can say, "Thanks, Mom and Dad, it feels great when you tell me I'm doing well on the Stoplight Diet."

When you praise your mom and dad, be sure to tell them exactly what they are doing that you like. What is so good about giving your parents praise is that it lets them know that you appreciate them, and that you are glad they are helping you stay on the Stoplight Diet.

Privileges

You may not know it, but praise is a type of reward for doing something good. Now that you have learned about praise, we are going to teach you about another kind of reward.

This reward is called a *privilege*. Everyone likes to get privileges, even your mom and dad.

What is a privilege? It's when your mother lets you stay up later than your usual bedtime. It's when you don't have to help clean up after dinner, even if it's your turn to do it. A privilege is when you get to have a party and it's not your birthday. It's when your mom and dad take you to an amusement park, or the beach, or a movie.

Privileges are special treats. They are things that do not happen every day. Starting right now, we are going to show you how you can earn privileges.

To earn privileges, you are going to make a special agreement with your mom and dad. This agreement will be written down on a piece of paper called a *contract*.

The contract will say that if you do certain things on the Stoplight Diet, your mom and dad will give you a certain privilege. The contract will tell you exactly what you have to do. It will also tell you exactly what privilege you can earn. But if you don't do what is in the contract, you will not earn the privilege.

Josh has had many contracts with his parents and has earned many privileges. He likes contracts because there are no surprises. The contract tells him exactly what he must do to earn the privilege. We think you will like that too. Here's how the Stoplight Diet contract works:

Your mom and dad will give you a piece of paper like the one shown on page 229. They will fill in your name, their names, and the date. Then they will write down what you must do to earn your privilege.

For instance, you might agree in the contract to write down your weight each morning and also to record everything that you eat during the day. In addition, you may agree to do both these things for at least five out of the next seven days. This is what Josh agreed to do in his first contract.

If you do what you agree to do in the contract, exactly as it is written, then you will earn the privilege. Your mom and dad will explain which privilege you can earn and will also write the privilege on the contract. They will also explain that if you don't write down your food and weigh yourself as agreed, then you will not earn the privilege. Finally, you and your mom and dad will all sign the contract.

The first week that Josh signed his contract, he did exactly what it said. He started working for his privilege on a Monday. His privilege would be to stay up an extra hour past his bedtime on the first Saturday after he met the contract.

On Monday, Josh wrote down everything he ate, and he weighed himself. He also recorded his weight (111 pounds) on the chart his mom and dad gave him.

Josh did the same thing on Tuesday. (He still weighed 111 pounds.)

Then, on Wednesday, Josh overslept and forgot to weigh himself. He was very worried that he would not earn his privilege. But he remembered that the contract said he had to do everything for five out of the next seven days. Even though he had missed one day, he could still do what he had agreed in the contract and earn his privilege.

On both Thursday and Friday, Josh weighed himself and wrote down all he ate. On Saturday morning, he got up early and weighed himself too. "I've only got one more day to go," he told his mom. "I think I'm going to make it." After breakfast and after lunch, Josh recorded what he ate.

On Saturday evening, Josh and his family went to a party at his aunt's house. They got back very late. Josh fell asleep in the car. When they got home, he went right to bed. It wasn't until Sunday morning that he remembered he had forgotten to write down what he ate for dinner at his aunt's.

"Oh no," Josh said to his dad. "I think I won't meet the contract." Josh felt like crying. He had worked so hard.

Josh's dad put his arm around Josh's shoulders. "Tell me why you think you won't meet the contract," he said. Josh explained. He told his dad how he had missed weighing himself on Wednesday.

"Okay," his dad said. "That counts as one day that you didn't meet the contract."

Then Josh told his dad how he had forgotten to write down what he ate for dinner on Saturday night.

"Okay," his dad said. "That makes two days that you didn't meet the contract. But the contract says that you must write down what you eat and weigh yourself five days out of seven. If you weigh yourself today and write down everything that you eat, you can still earn the privilege to stay up an extra hour."

"That's great!" Josh said. "I see how it works now. Thanks, Dad." Josh and his dad gave each other a big hug. Then Josh wrote down his weight (111 pounds again). He also carefully recorded what he ate all day long.

At the end of the day, he proudly showed his parents his Stoplight Diet habit book. "I did it!" he said with a big grin. "I met the contract and earned the privilege."

"You did a wonderful job of recording your weight and what you ate, Josh," his mother said.

"You sure did, Josh," said his father. "We're very proud of the way you kept at it."

"Thanks for helping me earn my privilege, Mom and Dad," Josh said.

You have learned something new this week. You now know how to make your parents feel good by giving them praise. You also know about privileges and contracts. You will get to use a contract this week. Maybe you will agree to keep track of your diet and your weight in your Stoplight Diet diary so that you can earn your privilege. Remember:

· Write the date at the top of each page.
· Record each food that you eat and say when you ate it.
· Write down how much food you eat.
· Always show whether a food is red (R), yellow (Y), or green (G).
· Remember to record the number of calories. To do this, look at the food guide in the back of the book.
· Put checkmarks in the boxes to show whether foods are proteins, grains, fruits and vegetables, or dairy.
· Record your weight every day on the chart your parents have given you.

Week 3 Quiz

Please answer true or false:

    1. Praise makes you feel good.   True   False
    2. Praise can also make your parents
feel good.   True   False
    3. You should never praise your parents.   True   False
    4. There are many times when you can praise your parents. Below, we have listed some times when it is a good idea to praise them. We also have included some times when

it is *not* a good idea to praise them. Circle the letters beside the times when it is a good idea to praise your parents.

    a. When they do not have red foods in the house.
    b. When they make nonfattening meals that taste good.
    c. When they buy red foods at the store.
    d. When they praise you for losing weight.
    e. When they go over your habit book with you.

    Jane is eight years old and is in the fourth grade. She and her family are losing weight on the Stoplight Diet, just like your family.

    Jane helps her mother pack lunch every day. Until her family started on the Stoplight Diet, Jane always put a small package of potato chips in her lunch bag. But last week, Jane helped her family get rid of all the red foods. There are no more potato chips in her house. Now, in place of potato chips, she packs the mini rice cakes her mom got at the supermarket. (Rice cakes are a low-calorie, yellow food.)

Answer true or false:

    5. One way Jane could thank her mother is by praising her for buying mini rice cakes instead of potato chips.   True   False

    6. Since the mini rice cakes are small, Jane does not need to write them on her food record form.   True   False

Answers

Remember, no fair peeking at the answers until you finish taking the quiz. Don't forget to show your answers to your parents. They will help you with anything you do not understand.

1. True
2. True
3. False
4. Circle *a, b, d* and *e*

5. True
6. False (You must always record everything that you eat.)

Week 4
Time to Exercise

This is your fourth week of the Stoplight Diet! You are becoming a real expert at losing weight. It must make you feel proud of yourself.

Josh felt proud of himself on the fourth week of the Stoplight Diet. Every morning he could hardly wait to wake up and see how much he weighed. Josh loved to watch the numbers on the scale go down. But most of all he liked getting on the scale knowing that he was no longer gaining weight.

During the first three weeks on the Stoplight Diet, Josh lost 1½ pounds. Kate also lost weight — about 2½ pounds during her first three weeks on the Stoplight Diet.

You too can expect to lose up to a pound a week if you keep to the calorie limit and eat no more than four red foods each week. Remember, if you eat fewer than four red foods a week, you will lose weight faster.

This week we are going to teach you how to speed up your weight loss with *exercise*. You already know that your body uses food as fuel. When you eat too much food, your body stores the extra as fat.

The more active you are, the more fuel your body uses. So the more exercise you do, the more fat (and calories) your body burns — provided, of course, that you do not overeat.

You don't have to do anything fancy to exercise. One of the best forms of exercise is walking. Josh loves to walk. He walks every day. Walking is one of the kinds of exercise that has helped him lose a total of 11 pounds. It's also what is helping him to stay slim.

Walking is an excellent exercise because it doesn't take any special equipment, except, of course, a comfortable pair of sneakers. You can walk all year round. You can walk by yourself or with someone else, but it is probably best — and it is certainly more fun — to walk with your parents, with your brother or sister, or with a friend.

Here is how Josh and his family use walking as an exercise. When Josh gets home from school, and when his mom and dad get home from work, they all go for a walk together. Usually they walk before dinner. But sometimes, if there isn't enough time, they will walk after dinner.

Josh and his family live near a park. They like to walk along a special exercise trail that runs through the park. They use the time not just to walk, but also to talk about what happened during the day at school and at work.

Josh and his parents began walking just 1 mile every day. It took them about half an hour. During that time, Josh's body burned fuel — about 69 calories. By walking every day, Josh burned an extra 483 calories a week (69 calories a day times 7 days a week equals 483 calories a week). That's more calories than he eats at one meal.

The next week, Josh and his parents tried to walk a little farther. They walked 1½ miles every day. On these walks, Josh burned 104 calories. During a week of walking every day, he burned 728 calories. That's about the number of calories Josh eats in two meals.

The third week, Josh and his parents walked 2 miles every day. Josh burned 138 calories. By walking every day, Josh burned 966 calories that week. Over a month, Josh burned enough calories to lose an extra pound!

Do you know what else happened? Josh found that he

started to have a lot more energy during the day. He also started to sleep a little better. He woke up in the morning feeling wide awake. Exercise made Josh's legs stronger. The more Josh and his parents walked, the firmer his legs got. They didn't feel as flabby or as fat. Josh knew that the exercise from walking helped to make his body healthier.

Josh also looked forward to spending the time with his parents every day on their walk. Josh's mom and dad work and have very busy schedules. Sometimes his mom has to work late. When that happens, Josh walks with his dad, who is usually home by five-thirty.

Josh really likes these walks with his parents. But at first he did not always want to go. Once, he even pouted and walked around with his head down. He was angry because he wanted to watch television and read his comic books instead of walking. But his parents wouldn't let him stay home.

His mom explained that sitting in front of the television burns very few calories. It doesn't help anyone lose weight. "You will lose weight a lot faster if you walk every day," his mother told him.

"You will also feel better, Josh," his dad said.

Josh went along, but he didn't like it very much. He even walked slowly on purpose. His parents didn't seem to notice. They just kept walking and talking and having fun. After a little while, Josh noticed that he did start to feel better. It felt good to be outside. He started to walk a little faster. Then he decided to jog a little. He caught up with his parents.

"Look at the stride you've got, Josh," his dad said. "You're going to be a really good runner."

Both his mom and his dad held out a hand to Josh. The three of them walked together, with Josh in the middle. "You know, Mom and Dad, I'm glad we came for a walk," Josh said.

"So are we," his parents said together.

We think that you will like walking with your mom and dad too. Of course, you don't always have to walk with your parents. Sometimes you may want to walk with a friend. If you have a dog, you might want to take him or her for a walk. Of course, always check with your parents first.

Kate also likes to walk every day. In the winter, Kate and her mom walk outdoors, even when it is cold. They put on layers of clothes and a coat. And they wear a hat, mittens, and waterproof boots.

On some very, very cold days, Kate's mom drives them to a nearby shopping mall. They go inside and walk around the mall. When they walk inside the mall, they don't need their heavy coats, mittens, or boots, because the mall is heated.

Kate and her mom time their walks. They make sure that they do not stop to shop. But they sometimes look in the windows as they walk by the stores. And they are very careful to avoid the restaurant area, where they might smell the aromas from the bakery that makes chocolate-chip cookies and fresh pie.

When it is very hot in the summer, Kate and her mom also go to the mall to walk because it is air-conditioned.

In fact, Kate and her mom are not the only people who walk in the mall. The mall owners now open the mall earlier and keep it open later so that people like Kate and her mom can use the mall to walk even when the stores aren't open.

Kate likes to look in the store windows for new clothes that she can buy now that she is slim. Before she lost so much weight, she used to have to shop in the chubby girls' department. Now she wears regular sizes and has lots of clothes from which to choose.

Kate has also started to take ballet lessons. She goes to class once a week. But Kate knows that exercising just once a week in ballet class is not enough to help her stay in shape or to lose more weight. She knows that she needs to burn calories exercising as often as possible. So she goes for a walk every day.

Like Kate, Josh does another form of exercise besides walking: he takes karate twice a week. Josh has already earned his green belt. Some day he wants to be a black belt.

You too can do other exercises. In fact, the more exercise you do, the better. Just remember that it is very important to start exercising slowly. If you do too much at first, you can injure yourself. Then you may have to wait a while to exercise again.

Jogging and running are activities that many of our young friends in the Stoplight Diet program like to do. Some children like to ride their bicycles. Others take up swimming. You can jump rope or roller-skate. It is also good to play games that involve a lot of running and moving around, such as soccer, football, basketball, and baseball. Ice skating, gymnastics, and tap dancing are other good exercises.

Whatever you do, each week it is important for you to burn a certain number of calories through exercise. Beginning this week, you will try to burn an extra 50 calories every day by exercising. You can do any exercise you want. But we suggest that you try walking. We think that you will like doing it as much as Josh and Kate do.

How many calories you burn during exercise depends on how much you weigh. It also depends on what kind of exercise you do and on how long you do it. Your mom or dad will use the exercise guide on pages 230 to 231 of this book to help you find out how many extra calories your body can burn by doing different kinds of exercise.

To help you lose weight, your mom and dad are going to include exercise as part of your weekly contract. How will this work?

To earn your privilege, you will probably agree to do several things:

· Weigh yourself every day.
· Eat 1,200 calories or less. (But remember, always eat at least 900 calories, and if you are six or seven years old, eat at least 1,000 calories a day.)
· Write down everything that you eat in your habit book.
· Eat no more than four red foods a week. (Remember, if you eat fewer than four red foods, you will lose weight faster.)
· Burn 50 extra calories a day by exercising. (If you already walk to school, or take ballet lessons, or do some other exercise activity, you must add a new exercise in addition to your present activity. This is because the amount of ex-

ercise you were doing when you started the Stoplight Diet was not enough to control your weight. You need more exercise to help you lose weight.)

To earn your privilege this week, you must do all the things in your contract *for the next five out of seven days.* It is also important to record in your habit book how long you exercise each day. Here is how Josh does it:

First, he turns to his daily exercise chart, finds the day of the week, and writes down the date. Then he writes down the kind of exercise he did. Next, he writes down how long he did the exercise and the number of extra calories he burned by doing it. (Your mom and dad will help you figure out how many calories you burn by exercising.) Josh's daily exercise chart for Week 4 of the Stoplight Diet is shown on page 156.

Two weeks from now, we want you to start burning 75 calories each day by exercising. Four weeks from now, we want you to burn 100 calories a day exercising. We will remind you of these goals later.

By exercising more, you will lose weight faster. You will also get in shape and become more fit. That will help you look and feel good. It also is very good for your health.

Josh and Kate learned that besides exercising more often there are many other things they can do to be more active and help burn more calories. Here are some of the things they do:

· Use the stairs instead of the elevator.
· Walk to and from school whenever possible. (They live close enough.)
· Walk to see friends who live nearby instead of having their mom or dad drive them.
· Ride a bicycle to the store or to do other errands (when they have their parents' permission).
· Walk or ride their bikes to their ballet or karate lessons.
· Watch television less. (Josh and Kate learned that they do not burn many calories by just sitting around in front of the television.)
· Play sports with friends as much as possible.

Name ___Josh_____ Week Number _4_

Calorie Goal: _50_ per day/_350_ per week

Day	Date	Type of Exercise	Time Spent Exercising (in minutes)	Number of Extra Calories Burned
Monday	Oct. 20	Walking (1 mile)	30	69
Tuesday	Oct. 21	Walking (1 mile)	30	69
Wednesday	Oct. 22	Walking (1 mile)	30	69
Thursday	Oct. 23	Walking (1 mile)	30	69
Friday	Oct. 24	Walking (1 mile)	30	69
Saturday	Oct. 25	Walking (1 mile)	30	69
Sunday	Oct. 26	Walking (1 mile)	30	69
			Total	483

Josh's Daily Exercise Chart

Now that you know some ways to be more active, see how you do on our quiz about exercise. Remember to show your answers to your mom and dad. And don't forget to have fun exercising!

Week 4 Quiz

Answer true or false:

1. Exercise will help you lose weight faster.   True   False
2. Exercise helps your body burn more calories.   True   False
3. Watching television burns a lot of calories.   True   False
4. Walking is a very good exercise to do.   True   False
5. Every day this week, it is important to burn 50 extra calories exercising.   True   False
6. Exercising once a week is enough to help you lose weight.   True   False
7. Using the stairs instead of the elevator is a good way to burn more calories.   True   False
8. Walking is a good exercise, but you must have lots of special equipment to do it.   True   False
9. It is important to write down how many calories you burn exercising every day.   True   False
10. Walking, jogging, soccer, swimming, and bicycle riding are exercises that burn a lot of calories.   True   False

Have your mom or dad help you with the next questions.

Kendra is twelve years old. She weighs 125 pounds. Here are the exercises that Kendra did this week:

Monday	Walked (at 2 miles per hour) for 20 minutes.
Tuesday	Forgot to exercise.
Wednesday	Walked (at 2 miles per hour) for 30 minutes.
Thursday	Rode her bicycle (at 5½ mph) for 30 minutes.
Friday	Walked (at 2 miles per hour) for 30 minutes.
Saturday	Walked (at 2 miles per hour) for 45 minutes.
Sunday	Played baseball for 60 minutes.

Use the chart below to fill out Kendra's exercise record for this week:

Day	Type of Exercise	Time Spent	Calories Burned
11. Monday	_____	_____	_____
12. Tuesday	_____	_____	_____
13. Wednesday	_____	_____	_____
14. Thursday	_____	_____	_____
15. Friday	_____	_____	_____
16. Saturday	_____	_____	_____
17. Sunday	_____	_____	_____

Answers

1. True	9. True	14. bicycling/30 minutes/126
2. True	10. True	
3. False	11. walking/20 minutes/60	15. walking/30 minutes/90
4. True		
5. True	12. none/none/none	16. walking/45 minutes/135
6. False		
7. True	13. walking/30 minutes/90	17. baseball/60 minutes/234
8. False		

Week 5
Set a
Good Example

Way to go! Here we are on the fifth week of the Stoplight Diet. You are doing an excellent job.

You are also setting a very good example for your parents. They are probably trying to lose weight too. Even if they don't need to lose weight, they are trying to eat in a healthier way — more green and yellow foods. They are trying to exercise more. They are trying to say "No thank you" to red foods.

Every time you stay within your calorie range, you set a good example for your parents. Every time you write down all the food you eat and show it to your parents, you remind them to write down everything that they eat. Each time you exercise, you help remind your mom and dad to exercise too. Every time you weigh yourself and write down how much you weigh in your daily habit book, you encourage them to do the same.

These are all ways that you set a good example for your parents. You also set a good example for your brothers and sisters. When you stick to the Stoplight Diet, you help yourself lose weight. And you help your family stay on the Stoplight Diet too.

At first, our friend Josh did not believe that he could

really be a good example for his mom and dad. But then Josh and his family went to visit his grandparents.

Josh's grandparents always have a lot of food in their house. His grandmother loves to cook. She bakes cookies and fresh cherry pie for Josh and his family.

"Grandma's kitchen is red food city," Josh says. Before their visit, Josh's family talked about how they could say "No thank you" to most of the red foods. Then, the whole week before they went, Josh and his mom, dad, and brother did not eat any red foods. That way they could eat four red foods while they visited Josh's grandparents.

Josh's mom also asked his grandparents to please not make as many red foods. "We have all worked very hard to lose weight," his mom said. "It would help us if you would not make any fattening foods."

Josh's grandmother listened. She made fewer red foods. But she said she had to make a few. She baked gingerbread cookies and only one cherry pie. (She usually baked two.)

For dessert one night, Josh's grandmother offered everyone a piece of the cherry pie with a scoop of ice cream on top.

Josh thought about the offer. Then he counted up the number of red foods he already had eaten at his grandparents' house: one Coke, one gingerbread cookie, and one piece of chocolate cake with a scoop of vanilla ice cream. That added up to four red foods.

"No thank you," Josh said when his grandmother asked if he wanted some cherry pie and ice cream. "I've already eaten four red foods this week." Josh's mother was standing nearby. She overheard what Josh said.

"You know, Josh, when I come here to visit, I am usually tempted to eat a lot of red foods," his mother said. "I was going to eat a piece of pie with ice cream, but I heard you say 'No thank you.' And you know what? It helped me say 'No thank you' too. I'm very proud of you."

Josh felt really good when his mother said that. It made him want to be a good example again for his mom and dad.

Our friend Kate also learned that she can set a good example for her parents. Kate's grandmother sent Kate's father a box of chocolates for his birthday. Each chocolate was shaped like a sailboat. Kate's dad loves to sail. So he was really pleased with his present. He also loves chocolate.

Since it was his birthday, Kate's dad offered to let each person in the family have some chocolate — even though chocolate is a red food.

Kate looked at the chocolate. It looked really good. But then Kate remembered the weight she had lost. She also thought about the weight she still wanted to lose, and she decided to say "No thank you" to the chocolate.

Kate's dad was really surprised. He knows how much Kate loves chocolate. "You know, Kate, you're right," he said. "You have reminded me that it's really better if I don't eat the chocolate either. I'll give it away tomorrow at my office. Thank you, Kate. I'm really glad about the way you helped me."

Kate gave her dad a hug.

Here are some of the ways that you can set a good example for your parents, just the way Kate and Josh did:

· Weigh yourself every day and record your weight.
· Say "No thank you" to red foods.
· Never eat more than 1,200 calories a day.
· Exercise as often as possible.
· As soon as possible after every meal, write down everything that you ate. (Remember: if you have any questions about a food, be sure to ask your mom or dad.)
· Try to eat slowly. It will help you eat less.
· Remember to praise your parents when they help you with the Stoplight Diet. Also praise them for trying to lose weight too.
· Thank your mom and dad for not having red foods in the house. Thank them, too, for not buying red foods at the store.
· Do things in front of your parents that will help to show them how to lose weight. For example, you can eat only green and yellow foods, or you might ask them to go walking with you. Also, cut back on how much television you watch. Remember that watching television burns very few calories.

When you lose weight on the Stoplight Diet, you help your parents lose weight too. And when your parents lose weight on our diet, their example helps remind you about losing weight. Your whole family can lose weight together.

Now that you know how to set a good example for your parents, please try our quiz.

Week 5 Quiz

Answer true or false:

1. Children can set a good example for their parents on the Stoplight Diet.　　　　True　False

2. When you exercise, you help remind your mom and dad to exercise too.　　　　True　False

3. Showing your food record to your mom and dad every day is a good way to remind them to fill out their food records too.　　　　True　False

4. Saying "No thank you" to red foods in front of your mom and dad helps them say "No thank you" to red foods too.　　　　True　False

5. When you weigh yourself every day, you help remind your mom and dad to weigh themselves too.　　　　True　False

6. Eating 1,200 calories or less every day does not help your mom or dad stay within the calorie limit too.　　　　True　False

7. When you lose weight, it helps your mom and dad lose weight too.　　　　True　False

8. Giving your mom and dad praise is a good way to help them stay with the Stoplight Diet.　　　　True　False

Sue and her mother are shopping at the grocery store. Sue sees her mom put a package of cookies in the grocery cart. She asks her mom if she may choose some fruit.

"That's a good idea," her mom says.

Sue chooses some beautiful green grapes. Then she picks some strawberries. Sue's mom watches as Sue does this. Then Sue's mom puts the cookies back and she picks up some oranges instead and puts them in the cart.

"Thanks, Mom," Sue says. "You made a really good choice."

Answer true or false:

9. Sue set a good example for her mom at the grocery store.   True   False

10. Sue's mom was reminded not to buy a red food (the cookies) when Sue asked to choose fruit.   True   False

Mark is ten years old. He is working very hard to lose weight on the Stoplight Diet. Mark weighs himself every morning before breakfast. Then he records his weight in his daily habit book.

Mark's father wants to lose weight too. But he has not been weighing himself every day. In fact, Mark's father is still gaining weight.

Mark wants to help his father. He makes sure that he weighs himself when his father is around. Mark also always tells his father when he has lost weight. Then he writes down what he weighs and shows his daily habit book to his dad.

Mark also watches his father carefully. When his father weighs himself, Mark says: "Thanks, Dad, for weighing yourself. It helps me remember to get on the scale too." Mark can tell that his father likes hearing that. Pretty soon, Mark's dad will be weighing himself every day too.

Answer true or false:

11. When Mark weighs himself every day, he helps remind his father to get on the scale too.   True   False

12. When Mark thanked his father for getting on the scale, he praised his dad.   True   False

13. Mark sets a good example for his
dad.   True   False

14. Mark's dad will probably lose less
weight when he starts weighing himself every
day.   True   False

Answers

Remember to show your answers to your mom and dad.
You can help set a good example by reminding them to read
their chapter and answer their quiz questions.

1. True	6. False	11. True
2. True	7. True	12. True
3. True	8. True	13. True
4. True	9. True	14. False
5. True	10. True	

Week 6
Keep to the
Stoplight Signals

You now know about nutrition and how to eat good food from the Basic Four food groups. You know about exercising. You know about keeping track of how much you weigh. You know about red, yellow, and green foods and how to stay in your calorie range. You know how to lose weight.

Are you surprised about how much you have learned? Our friend Josh was. He was also surprised at the weight he lost. Josh lost almost 4 pounds by the sixth week of the Stoplight Diet.

Kate did well at losing weight too. By the sixth week, Kate had also lost 4 pounds. But she was a little discouraged. During the first four weeks, Kate lost weight pretty fast. Each week, she lost about a pound.

But during the fifth week, Kate did not lose any weight, even though she did everything the same. Kate wondered what was wrong. She ate the same amount of calories. She exercised the same way. She wrote down her food. She weighed herself every day. She didn't snack. She didn't even eat any red foods that week!

But then Kate learned that sometimes during a diet, your weight stays steady. This is called a *plateau* ("pla-toe"). It means something that is level or that stays the same.

No one knows exactly why a plateau occurs. But it does end. (Kate's plateau was over by Week 7, when her weight started to go down again.) So if your weight stays the same for a little while — if it is at a plateau — don't worry. It is very important to stay on the Stoplight Diet during a plateau or if your weight goes up a little. Sometimes it also helps if you do a little more exercise.

This week, we want you to increase the amount of exercise you do — whether your weight stays steady or not. Every day, you need to burn *75 extra calories* by exercising. These extra calories will help you lose weight faster. The exercise will also help you get in shape.

During the fifth week, Josh began karate. He went just two times that week, but in the sixth week, he began going three times a week. He really liked what he learned. Josh also continued his walks with his mom and dad. He was able to burn 90 calories more a day by walking 20 minutes longer.

Kate tried something new too in the fifth week. She began to take ballet. Kate had always wanted to be a dancer. But until she went on the Stoplight Diet, she was afraid people would laugh at her when she wore her leotard. By the sixth week she had lost 4 pounds, and she couldn't wait to go to ballet class in her new pink leotard.

Perhaps you want to try some new kind of exercise. This is a good time to talk about it with your mom and dad. Why not suggest that part of this week's contract include one beginning lesson in a new activity? Josh did that when he wanted to try karate. He was not sure he would like it, so his dad arranged for him to go to one karate class.

After the class, Josh knew that he wanted to take karate. So, Josh's dad signed him up for more lessons. Now Josh has his green belt and is on his way to one day earning a black belt.

Josh and Kate also learned something else during the sixth week of the Stoplight Diet. They learned how to stick with the diet program.

The Secret of Self-Control

You know by now that there are many chances to slip off the Stoplight Diet. You have to be strong in saying "No thank you" to red foods. We know that you do that.

You also need to exercise regularly. We know that you do that too.

But we also know that it is sometimes tough to be around your friends when they are eating red foods. Do you remember how Kate said "No thank you" to ice cream when her friend Julie offered her some?

That took a lot of *self-control* from Kate. Self-control is what you use when you eat no more than 1,200 calories a day. It's what you use to say no to red foods. Self-control is using the new behaviors you have learned to do something hard. By making it to the sixth week of the Stoplight Diet, you have shown that you have a lot of self-control.

This week we want to teach you some hints that will help you have even stronger self-control. We taught these same lessons to Josh and Kate. The lessons helped them very much. We think they will help you too.

Josh is very lucky. He has a friend named Scott who has never made fun of Josh's weight. When Josh told Scott that he was going on a diet, Scott did not laugh. He said: "That's great, Josh. I hope you do very well."

Scott also asked Josh some questions about the Stoplight Diet. Josh told Scott about the red, the yellow, and the green foods. He told Scott about walking every day.

"I like to go for walks too," Scott said. "If you ever want someone to walk with, I'd like to go along."

Josh knew then what a good friend Scott is. Friends are very important. They can help you on the Stoplight Diet or they can make the Stoplight Diet very difficult for you.

Josh also has a friend named Alex. Alex is not very helpful to Josh. He always offers Josh food that he knows Josh is not supposed to eat. Josh always says, "No thank you, Alex." But sometimes Josh must use a lot of self-control to say no. Especially when Alex offers chocolate-chip cookies.

"Oh, come on, Josh, have just one," Alex always says. But Josh never does.

Alex is also one of the people who made fun of Josh when he was fat. "Look at you, Josh," Alex used to say. "You are really tubby." Then Alex would laugh.

Now that Josh has lost weight, Alex doesn't make fun of how fat he is anymore. Instead, he teases Josh about being on a diet.

"How's your diet going, Josh?" Alex likes to yell across the schoolyard so that everyone can hear. "Let's go get some ice cream," Alex also likes to say. "Josh, can you have ice cream?" As you can see, Alex can be very mean.

Josh used to get upset when Alex acted this way. But when he got upset, Alex only got meaner.

Now, Josh knows how to handle him. He learned what to say to Alex as part of the Stoplight Diet.

When Alex says in front of everyone, "How's your diet going, Josh?" Josh now says: "Great. I'm feeling healthier by the day."

Josh has learned not to be embarrassed by Alex's teasing. He knows that if he lets what Alex says bother him, then he gives Alex what he wants.

Now when Alex teases Josh for not being able to eat red foods, Josh says, "I'm proud of myself for sticking to my diet, Alex!"

When Alex says, "Josh was so fat that now he's on a diet to lose weight," Josh says: "Yes, Alex, I was overweight. That's why it's so great that I'm changing my eating habits and losing weight."

Josh also sometimes tells Alex, "I am trying to lose weight so that I can look and feel better."

When Alex used to tease Josh, most of the other children would laugh. But now, when Josh responds to Alex's teasing, very few people laugh. Many of them even come to Josh's defense. One boy said: "Leave him alone, Alex. Don't you have anything better to do?" And another friend told Alex, "You know, Alex, you could stand to lay off some of the candy bars yourself." Josh likes it a lot that his friends come to his defense. But even if no one defends him, Josh knows that he is no longer bothered by Alex. That makes Josh feel good about himself.

Just the Right Words

Do you ever get teased by other children? You can do what Josh did. Here's how he practiced. Josh stood in front of the mirror and pretended he was talking to Alex. He imagined looking Alex right in the eye. He used a very firm voice — not loud, but strong. Then he practiced what he was going to say to Alex.

You can do this too. Your mom and dad can probably help you think of other things to say to children who tease you or give you a hard time about the Stoplight Diet. Give it a try. We think you will be pleased with the results.

Josh found out that the best way to keep his self-control strong is to be prepared with just the right answers.

Now when a friend says, "Here, have some potato chips," Josh says, "No thanks, I'm not eating those these days."

If one of his buddies says, "Let's go get an ice-cream cone," Josh says, "I'd rather go to the comic-book store." Other times, Josh invites the friend home to have a frozen fruit-juice bar. (Josh's mother makes these and keeps them in the freezer. Maybe your mom or dad could too.) Josh says: "I'll treat. You can save your money. We'll get fruit bars at my house."

Friends Can Help

When Josh is visiting a friend and the friend says, "My mom will give us some cake and then we can go shoot some hoops," Josh says: "I'm not eating cake these days. Have you got some fruit? Or, would your mom let us make some popcorn?"

At Scott's house, Josh never has to worry. Scott understands what Josh can't eat. He always has low-calorie drinks for Josh. He never offers red foods. Scott even asks his mom not to add butter to Josh's food if Josh comes over for dinner.

Scott also goes for walks with Josh. Do you have a friend

who helps you with the Stoplight Diet? If you do, you are very lucky.

Always make sure that you praise your friend for helping you. By praising your friend, you will make your friend want to help you again.

Maybe you have a good friend who hasn't thought about doing some of the things that Scott does to help Josh. If so, you can ask that friend to help you stay on the Stoplight Diet. Tell your friend what kind of help you would like to have. Explain about red, yellow, and green foods. When you do this, be sure to look your friend right in the eye. This way, your friend knows that you feel what you are saying is very important.

Kate asked her friend Elizabeth to help her with the Stoplight Diet. Kate explained to Elizabeth what a red food is. "Red foods are very fattening," Kate said. "They have lots of calories. If I eat too many calories, I will gain weight. Sometimes, it's hard, because I like red foods. Cake and candy and chocolate-chip cookies are red foods. So is fried chicken and soda pop. Elizabeth, would you please help me by not eating red foods when I am around?" Kate asked.

"Sure, Kate," Elizabeth said.

The next time Kate played at Elizabeth's house, Elizabeth's mom offered some ice cream. "Mom," Elizabeth said, "could we please have some fruit instead, because Kate is trying to lose weight."

Elizabeth's mom put the ice cream away and cut up some strawberries. She gave them to the girls.

"Thanks a lot, Elizabeth, for helping me," Kate said.

Elizabeth smiled. "You're welcome, Kate," she said.

Learning New Tricks

Kate and Josh learned two more "tricks" to help themselves use self-control and stay on the Stoplight Diet. Here they are:

• *Promise yourself a reward time if you stick to the Stoplight Diet.* One way to do this is to say to yourself, "If I don't eat any red foods today, I'll give myself a reward." You could reward yourself by reading an extra chapter of your favorite book at bedtime. You could wear your favorite clothes to school tomorrow as a reward for you sticking with your plan. You could arrange for a friend to come over as your reward, but always remember to ask your mom or dad first.

When you have thought of a reward for doing something on the Stoplight Diet, never give yourself the reward unless you have really earned it.

· *If you feel a very strong urge to have a red food, do something else right away.* Josh sometimes feels that he wants a red food very badly. He says it is like having a mountain lion breathing down his neck. Josh can feel the mountain lion standing there. It is very hard to forget.

When that happens, Josh tells himself that he will *not* eat a red food. Then he does something else right away to forget about the red food. He rides his bicycle around the block or takes a walk with his brother. Josh tells us that in a little while, the mountain lion has turned into a big pussycat. And you know what? He doesn't want the red food anymore. We think Josh's trick will work for you too. Be sure to congratulate yourself when you use it!

Now that you know about self-control and about how to ask your friends for help, try this week's quiz. It starts on the next page. Show your answers to your mom and dad. Ask them to help you practice some good things to say to children who tease you about your weight or about the Stoplight Diet. And don't forget: Increase the amount of calories you burn this week. Try to burn 75 calories extra every day.

Week 6 Quiz

Answer true or false:

1. Friends can help you lose weight on the Stoplight Diet.   True   False

2. If someone teases you about your weight, it is best not to get upset.   True   False

3. It is a good idea to practice what to say to people who tease you about being on a diet.   True   False

4. Self-control is something you learn to do that helps you stay within 1,200 calories a day and helps you say "No thank you" to red foods.   True   False

5. If a really good friend has done something to help you on the Stoplight Diet, you don't need to say thanks.   True   False

6. When you have a friend who often offers you red foods, it is a good idea to prepare an answer ahead of time.   True   False

7. When you ask someone to help you with the Stoplight Diet, you do not have to look the person in the eye.   True   False

8. When other children know that you are serious about losing weight, they will not bother you so much.   True   False

Polly is nine years old. She has been on the Stoplight Diet for the last six weeks. Polly is doing very well. She has lost 3 pounds so far.

Each day at lunch, Polly chooses to drink skim milk. But Peggy, one of her classmates, teases Polly about being on a diet and drinking skim milk.

Polly decides to think of things to say to Peggy. She asks her mom for help. Then Polly practices in front of the mirror at home what she will say when Peggy teases her.

Here are some of the things that Polly could say:

  a. "Peggy, I'm proud of myself for sticking to my diet. Skim milk is good to drink and it helps me lose weight."
  b. "Peggy, you're so mean. I don't like you anymore."
  c. "Peggy, I'm trying to lose weight so I can look and feel better. Drinking skim milk helps me do that."
  d. "Peggy, I've been overweight. That's why it is so great that I am changing my eating habits. Drinking skim milk is one of the ways I'm doing that."

9. Write down the letter that's next to each thing it would be good for Polly to say to Peggy.

10. Which one would probably not be a good idea to say because it will show Peggy that she has made Polly feel upset?

Answers

1. True	5. False	8. True
2. True	6. True	9. a, c, d
3. True	7. False	10. b
4. True		

Week 7
Remember
the Rules

By now, the seventh week, you are an expert at the Stoplight Diet. If you are like our friends Josh and Kate, you know which foods are red, yellow, and green. Both Josh and Kate also know many of the calorie counts by heart. Josh's dad likes to rely on Josh's knowledge. (He is really proud of what Josh has learned.)

Sometimes, after dinner, when Josh's family is filling out their food habit books, Josh's dad will ask Josh for help in writing down calories. "How many calories in half a cup of brown rice?" Josh's dad says.

"Eighty calories, Dad," Josh says with a smile.

"How many calories in three ounces of baked chicken?" Josh's dad asks.

"One hundred and fifty calories, Dad," Josh says patiently.

"How many calories in half a cup of broccoli?" Josh's dad asks.

"Twenty calories, Dad," Josh says, grinning.

"You sure know your calories, Josh," his dad says. Josh can tell his dad is impressed.

Josh and his family know that it takes work to lose weight. They also know that if they are going to keep losing weight —

and make sure that they don't gain any weight back — they must plan ahead.

Here are some of the things that Josh and his family do. We think that these tips will help you and your family too.

• *Eat only at the table in your kitchen (or dining room or breakfast room)*. Josh and his mom and dad learned that if you eat in many different places in your house, you will be tempted to eat more often.

For instance, if you usually eat in front of the television in the living room, then every time you watch television, you will think about eating. If you eat when you play a game in the den, then every time you play the game you will think about eating. The same thing happens if you eat while you are in bed, or while you read, or while you do anything else. It's best to eat only at the table.

Josh and his family always pay attention when they eat. They never read at the table. And when dinner is finished, they clear the dishes right away so that they will not be tempted to eat more.

• *Keep red foods out of the house for good.* Even after Josh and his family lost all the weight they needed to lose, they still did not bring red foods into their house. They know that if the red foods are around, they will eat them. If they eat red foods again, they will gain back the weight they have lost.

• *Always eat three meals a day.* When you skip meals, you can get very hungry. Then there is a danger that you will overeat. It is best to eat three meals every day. Each meal should be about 350 calories.

• *Try to eat small portions.* At Josh's house, his mom and dad realized that when big bowls of food are put on the table, their family eats much more food. So Josh's parents started serving food in the kitchen. They put small portions on each plate, because they have learned that when you finish what's on your plate you feel full, no matter how much or how little you have eaten.

• *Exercise regularly.* The more active you are, the faster

you will lose weight. Exercise also helps keep the weight off for good. Josh tries to exercise at about the same time every day. Usually at about five P.M., Josh and his mom and dad take a walk. Now everyday at five P.M., Josh thinks about exercise.

Also, three times a week, Josh goes to karate. Josh also walks to and from school. He tries to walk up and down stairs whenever he can rather than riding an elevator. Some days, he also rides his bike after school.

Josh also tries to keep things around that will help him remember to exercise. He keeps a ball on a shelf in his room where he can see it. His baseball glove is nearby. Josh subscribes to a sports magazine that also helps him remember to be more active.

But Josh is careful never to overdo exercise. He knows that if he injures himself, or if his muscles get very sore, he will have to stop exercising for a while. So he is careful and does not overdo exercise.

· *Limit the amount of television you watch.* When Josh and his family started the Stoplight Diet, they added up all the hours they spent watching television. To do this, Josh, his brother, and his mom and dad kept a piece of paper, a pencil, and a clock near the television. For one week, Josh and his family watched TV just as they usually did. The only difference was that they wrote down on the paper how much time they spent doing it.

Were they surprised at the end of the week! They found out that they watched about 3 hours of television every weekday night. On weekends, they watched about 4 hours a day. The total for the week was 23 hours. That meant that Josh and his family spent almost 24 hours — a whole day — every week watching television.

Of course, watching television once in a while can be fun. But when you are trying to lose weight, or to keep off the weight that you have lost, television does not help — unless you are watching an exercise show or a special program on nutrition. As you know, you burn very few calories while you sit in front of the television.

To help stay more active, Josh and his family agreed to

watch no more than one hour of television a day. This way they don't miss their *very* favorite shows. They watch less television and exercise more.

Try keeping track of how much you and your family watch television in one week. See if you can cut back on how much you watch. These changes will help you lose weight and stay slim.

· *Offer to take low-calorie snacks to a party.* If a friend invites him to a party, Josh sometimes pops a big batch of popcorn and takes it along. Other times he takes a bowl of grapes. He has also gone with graham crackers and pretzels and frozen fruit-juice bars. (Not all at once, of course!) Josh likes to share his low-calorie snacks with everyone at the party.

· *Plan ahead for holidays and other special occasions.* Josh and his parents know that there are always going to be times when it is very hard to stick to the Stoplight Diet. Christmas is one of those times. So is Easter. Thanksgiving can be tough too. There are birthdays, anniversaries, and parties. Here's what Josh does about holidays.

The week before a holiday or special occasion, he is especially careful about how much he eats. During this week, Josh eats no red foods. He knows that there will probably be many red foods during the holiday or special occasion. He is also even more careful about eating no more than 1,200 calories each day.

On the day of the special occasion, Josh eats a small breakfast and a small lunch. That way, he is able to eat some extra calories at the special meal or party and still stay within his daily limit.

At the party or special meal, Josh tries to have only one or two bites of a red food, a very small portion at most — such as half a piece of birthday cake, or two spoonfuls of ice cream, or only one Christmas-tree cookie.

Once Josh is finished eating, he asks if he may be excused from the table. He tries to keep away from the food. Lots of times, he goes outside for a walk after having a big meal.

Josh and his parents never have second portions of yellow or red foods. (It's okay to have seconds of green foods.)

They also never take home red-food leftovers. But they are always polite when they refuse these foods.

The Art of Self-Control

Whenever Josh is in a place where there are many red foods, he remembers the secret of self-control. Self-control is what you use to solve certain problems. It helps you to do something hard all by yourself.

Here is what Josh does when he faces a tough situation that will make him want to eat more than he should. First, he gets a piece of paper and a pencil. Then he writes down these four questions (he leaves space after each question for his answer):

1. *What is my problem?*
2. *What is my plan?*
3. *Did I stick to my plan?*
4. *How did I do?*

Here's how Josh filled out his paper when he knew he was going to be at a friend's birthday party where there would be many tempting red foods.

Under *"What is my problem?"* Josh wrote:

Going to a birthday party where there will be many red foods.

Under *"What is my plan?"* Josh wrote three things. Here they are:

A. *I will look at all the red foods very carefully. Then I will pick out my favorite one.*
B. *I will eat only that one red food.*
C. *I will ask Mrs. Brandon to give me only half a portion of that food.*

By having a written plan, Josh knew that he could use self-control to avoid eating too many red foods. During the party, he remembered the third question: *"Did I stick to my plan?"* This helped him not to overeat while he was there. When cake and ice cream were served, Josh asked that he be given only cake. "May I please have just a small piece?" he asked. Josh was doing a good job of sticking to his plan.

After the party, Josh checked to see how he did. "I did really well," he told his mom and dad. "I ate only one red food — the birthday cake — and I asked for a small piece." Page 180 shows what Josh's written plan for self-control looked like when he was finished with it.

Sometimes, Josh comes home and finds that he didn't do very well at sticking to his plan during a special occasion. Then he talks about it with his mom and dad. Together they help him figure out how he can do better the next time.

Josh's mother always reminds him of something very important: If once in a while Josh slips and eats more than he should, it doesn't mean that he has failed at the Stoplight Diet. "Everyone can have a bad day, Josh," his mother tells him. "What's important is to figure out how you can help avoid a bad day the next time. It's also very, very important for you to go right back on the Stoplight Diet tomorrow. Even though you had trouble today, I am still very proud of what you have done until now."

By now you really have learned a lot. You should be proud of yourself. This week's quiz starts on page 181. It tests what you know about self-control and staying on the Stoplight Diet. Don't forget to show your parents your answers. Also, be sure to ask them any questions you may have. Good luck!

1. <u>What is my problem?</u>
   Going to a birthday party where there will be many red foods.

2. <u>What is my plan?</u>
   A. I will look at all the red foods very carefully. Then I will pick out my favorite one.
   B. I will eat only that one red food.
   C. I will ask Mrs. Brandon to give me only a small portion of that food.

3. <u>Did I stick to my plan?</u>
   Yes. I asked for just one red food — a small piece of chocolate cake (my favorite).

4. <u>How did I do?</u>
   Great! I ate only one red food and had just half a piece.

Josh's Self-Control Plan

Week 7 Quiz

Answer true or false:

1. You should always eat three meals
a day.   True   False

2. It's okay to keep a few red foods in
the house.   True   False

3. People on the Stoplight Diet need
to plan ahead to reduce the chance of eating too many red foods on a special oc-
casion.   True   False

4. Watching less television will help you
stay active and lose more weight.   True   False

5. It's okay to eat in any room of your
house.   True   False

6. Eating small portions and serving
those portions from the kitchen helps you
eat less.   True   False

7. During special occasions, it is a good
idea to ask to be excused from the table
when you are finished eating so that you
do not eat too much.   True   False

8. When you know you will be tempted
by a lot of red foods, you should think up
a written plan to strengthen your self-
control.   True   False

Margaret is eleven years old. She has been invited to a
birthday party. Margaret knows there will be a lot of red
foods at the party. So the week before the party, she does
not eat any red foods. She also exercises a little extra and
she makes sure that she does not eat more than 1,200 calories
a day.

On the day of the party, Margaret eats a small breakfast.
To help her self-control, she also writes down the same four
questions that Josh uses. Margaret already knows what her
problem is: she might eat too many red foods at the party.
She decides that her plan will be to eat just one small portion

of a red food. At the party, Margaret is offered a big piece of chocolate cake with a scoop of ice cream on top.

9. Which of the following choices should Margaret make?

   a. Eat the cake and the ice cream to be polite and ask for more.
   b. Ask if she could please have a small piece of cake without the ice cream.
   c. Give back the fattening cake and ask for three large scoops of ice cream instead.

As the children are leaving the party, each partygoer is offered a piece of cake to take home.

10. What should Margaret say?

   a. "No thank you. I really liked the cake, but I have had enough."
   b. "Thank you very much. I would love to take a piece home to eat."
   c. "Don't forget to give me enough for my mom and dad too."

Answers

1. True
2. False
3. True
4. True
5. False
6. True
7. True
8. True
9. b
10. a

Week 8
Stay Trim
and Healthy Forever

Congratulations! You've done it. You've made it to the eighth week of the Stoplight Diet.

This week, you will learn all the rest of what we want to teach you. You already know how to lose weight. You have become a master at nutrition, the study of foods. And you know how to exercise. In fact, as one of our last instructions, we want you to begin burning *100 extra calories a day by exercising*. That will be double the amount since you first started to exercise more. You have done a great job!

This is the last chapter that you will read in *The Stoplight Diet* book, but it is not the end of the program. The most important part is still to come.

As we just said, you now know how to lose weight. Losing weight is one part of the Stoplight Diet. The next part, the most important one, is keeping off the weight forever. That's what we are going to teach you this week.

Of course, before you start to work on keeping off the weight forever, you must first have reached your goal weight. This is the weight that you set with your mom and dad in the first week of the Stoplight Diet.

It takes most children on the Stoplight Diet more than eight weeks to reach their goal weight. Josh got to his goal weight after four months on the Stoplight Diet. Kate got to hers after six months. It does not matter how long it takes you to get there. The most important thing is to do it. Don't quit until you reach your goal weight. We know you will be very happy when you do.

When you reach your goal weight, you will want to keep your new, slim figure. Here is how to do it:

· *For a week or two after you reach your goal weight, keep eating 1,200 calories a day.* Your mom and dad will then show you how to add calories slowly each week.

· *Weigh yourself every day.* It will be very important during this time to weigh yourself. If you gain any weight, you must stop eating some of the extra calories. Your mom and dad will tell you more about this when the time comes.

· *Every six months, check to see if you need a new goal weight.* Your mom and dad can show you how to use a table at the back of this book to check whether your height and weight are average. You probably will need their help to read this table. As you grow older, you will grow taller. You will also gain weight as you become taller. That's okay. In fact, that's what you are supposed to do. What you and your mom and dad need to check is that you don't gain too much weight. If you do, they will help you set a new goal weight.

· *Keep red foods out of the house.* When red foods are in the house, you and your family will eat them. It's that simple. And if you start eating red foods again, you will gain more weight than you should. We don't want that to happen to you. We're sure you don't want it to happen either. So keep the red foods out of the house.

· *Never eat more than four red foods a week.* You know how fattening red foods are. They have a lot of fat and sometimes a lot of sugar. It's not healthful to eat too much fat or sugar. So limit the number of red foods you eat each week to four or less. Doing that will help you keep the weight off for good.

· *Keep writing in your habit book.* Once you have reached your goal weight, you don't have to write down everything you eat for the rest of your life. Instead of writing down what you eat every day, choose one week a month to record everything that you eat. Carefully measure or weigh all your food during that week. Check to be sure that you are following all the rules you learned on the Stoplight Diet. Make some changes if you find that you are straying far from the way you should eat on the Stoplight Diet.

For instance, if you are eating too many calories each day, cut back for a while to no more than 1,200 a day. If you are not eating a balanced diet, reread "Week 2: The ABCs of Smart Eating," review the Basic Four food groups, and start eating the right number of servings from each group every day. You may also find that you are eating larger portions of food. In that case, go back to measuring your food carefully each day.

· *Set a weight limit.* Your mom and dad will help you set a limit once you reach your goal weight. If you gain weight and reach this limit, don't eat more than 1,200 calories a day until you lose 2 or 3 pounds and get back to your goal weight. The weight limit helps you make sure that you never gain too much weight again. Check your weight limit every six months. As you grow, it will need to be raised. Ask your mom and dad to help you figure out your new weight limit.

· *Exercise regularly.* It's best if you keep exercising every day. The more active you stay, the less chance you have of gaining weight. Exercise also helps your body stay healthy.

· *Keep planning ahead for special occasions or holidays.* Having a celebration does not mean that you can eat anything or everything that you want. Remember the four-red-foods rule. Eat only small portions of red foods. If you can, try to just have a bite.

· *Make "kitchen checks" every few months with your mom and dad.* Look in the cupboards to see if any red foods have crept back in your house. Don't forget to check the refrigerator and the freezer too.

· *If you gain a little bit of weight, don't worry.* Gaining back some weight is called a *relapse.* A relapse, or return of some weight, can happen to anyone. If it happens to you, go right back on the Stoplight Diet. Get your mom and dad to help you again. Exercise more. Write down everything that you eat. Measure your food. Count calories. Limit red foods. You can keep your weight in balance. You now know how to do it.

Josh and Kate are keeping their weight in check. Josh has already earned his blue belt in karate. He is well on his way to earning his black belt. What Josh likes about his new figure is that he can move much faster in karate class. His kicks are higher, and he can dodge his sparring partner much better than he could when he was fat. Josh's karate instructor, Master Choy, has also noticed how much faster Josh can move since he lost weight. Master Choy is very proud of Josh's progress and tells him so. That makes Josh feel very good.

Kate is doing more and more ballet. She noticed as she lost weight that she could pirouette much more gracefully than she had before. Kate loves looking at herself now in the ballet class mirrors. Yet even a year ago, Kate was embarrassed to watch herself as she tried to follow her ballet teacher's instructions.

Both Josh and Kate have become more interested in clothes. "It's fun to go shopping now that I don't have to buy clothes in the husky department," Josh says.

Are Josh and Kate happy that they worked so hard on the Stoplight Diet? "I wouldn't go back to being fat for anything in the world," Kate says.

"Neither would I," agrees Josh. "I just feel so much better about myself now.

"And now I've got a couple of friends who are trying to lose weight too," Josh says, with a proud smile. "I plan on helping them, now that I'm a Stoplight Diet expert."

Week 8 Quiz

This is our last quiz. Don't forget to discuss your answers with your mom and dad. They will continue to help you on the Stoplight Diet. And be sure to ask them any questions that you may have.

You have really worked hard. Keep at it. Like Josh and Kate, you now belong to a very special group of people. Remember, you have successfully learned the Stoplight Diet. Keep giving a green light to your good health!

Answer true or false:

1. Weighing yourself every day is a very good way to help make sure that you don't gain any weight.   True   False

2. Now that you are thinner, you can go off the Stoplight Diet and eat anything that you want.   True   False

3. Once you reach your goal weight, you can eat as many red foods as you want.   True   False

4. Losing weight is important, and so is keeping it off.   True   False

5. If you start to gain some weight, you need to start writing in your habit book again right away.   True   False

6. When you reach your goal weight, you no longer need to plan ahead for holidays or special occasions.   True   False

7. Exercise is very important for continuing to lose weight and for keeping the weight off for good.   True   False

Twelve-year-old Sam lost 15 pounds on the Stoplight Diet over four months. Sam is very proud of his new, slim look. His parents tell him what a good job he did. His grandparents think he looks terrific.

Now that Sam has reached his goal weight, he no longer

thinks that he has a weight problem. He has stopped weighing himself every day. He now eats a lot more than he did when he went on the Stoplight Diet. When he goes to his grandparents' house, they give him lots of red foods.

Answer yes or no:

8. Sam thinks that he is finished for-ever with dieting. Is he right? Yes No

9. Should Sam be eating any food he wants to eat now? Yes No

10. Should Sam still limit his red foods to no more than four a week? Yes No

11. Sam has stopped weighing himself every day. Is this a good idea? Yes No

12. If Sam follows the Stoplight Diet rules for keeping weight off, will he stay more trim and healthy? Yes No

Answers

1. True	5. True	9. No
2. False	6. False	10. Yes
3. False	7. True	11. No
4. True	8. No	12. Yes

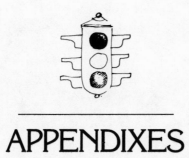

APPENDIXES

Appendix A: Ideal-Weight Tables

BOYS' IDEAL BODY WEIGHTS (IN POUNDS)

Height (in inches)	Age (in years)												
	6	7	8	9	10	11	12	13	14	15	16	17	18
38	33												
39	34												
40	35												
41	37	37											
42	38	38	38										
43	38	41	40										
44	43	43	43										
45	45	45	45	45									
46	47	48	47	47									
47	49	50	49	49	49								
48	52	52	52	52	52								
49	54	54	54	54	54	54							
50		57	57	57	57	57	57						
51		60	60	60	60	60	60						
52		62	63	63	63	63	63	63					
53			66	66	65	65	67	67					
54			68	68	69	68	69	69	70				
55			71	71	72	72	72	73	73				
56				75	75	76	76	77	77	78			
57				78	79	80	80	82	82	82			
58					82	83	84	84	85	85			
59					86	87	87	88	88	89	89		
60						90	91	92	93	94	96		
61						94	95	96	97	98	101	105	
62						99	100	101	103	103	107	111	116
63							106	105	107	108	111	115	120
64							109	110	111	113	115	119	124
65								114	116	118	120	125	129
66								117	121	123	126	129	132
67									127	127	131	134	136
68									131	132	135	139	141
69									135	136	138	141	144
70									140	142	143	145	147
71										146	147	148	150
72										149	152	154	156
73										153	156	159	161

SOURCE: World Health Organization

NOTES: To find ideal weights for children under six or for those who fall outside the height ranges shown, consult your physician. For individuals aged nineteen or older, use the adults' table.

GIRLS' IDEAL BODY WEIGHTS (IN POUNDS)

Height (in inches)	Age (in years)												
	6	7	8	9	10	11	12	13	14	15	16	17	18
39	34												
40	35	35											
41	37	37											
42	38	38											
43	40	40	40										
44	42	42	42										
45	45	44	45										
46	47	46	47	47	47								
47	50	50	49	50	50								
48	51	52	52	52	52	52							
49	53	53	54	55	55	56							
50		56	57	58	58	60	60						
51		59	60	60	61	62	62						
52		63	63	63	64	64	66						
53			66	67	67	67	68	70					
54			68	70	70	71	71	73					
55				73	74	74	75	77	78				
56				76	78	78	79	80	84				
57					81	82	82	84	89	93			
58					84	87	86	88	93	96	100		
59					87	91	90	93	97	101	104	105	
60						95	96	97	101	105	108	109	111
61						97	101	101	105	108	112	113	114
62							105	106	108	112	114	115	116
63							110	111	112	115	116	118	118
64							114	115	117	118	120	121	122
65								120	120	121	124	125	126
66								124	125	126	128	128	131
67								127	129	131	133	133	134
68									131	133	134	136	138
69									133	135	136	138	140
70									134	136	138	140	141

SOURCE: World Health Organization

NOTES: To find ideal weights for children under six or for those who fall outside the height ranges shown, consult your physician. For individuals aged nineteen or older, use the adults' table.

ADULTS' IDEAL BODY WEIGHTS
(AGES 25 AND OVER)

MEN

Height			Ideal Weight
Ft.	In.	Total Inches	(in pounds)
5	1	61	123.5
5	2	62	127
5	3	63	130
5	4	64	133
5	5	65	136.5
5	6	66	140.5
5	7	67	145
5	8	68	149
5	9	69	153
5	10	70	157
5	11	71	162
6	0	72	166.5
6	1	73	171
6	2	74	176
6	3	75	181

WOMEN

Height			Ideal Weight
Ft.	In.	Total Inches	(in pounds)
4	8	56	101.5
4	9	57	104
4	10	58	107
4	11	59	110
5	0	60	113
5	1	61	116
5	2	62	119.5
5	3	63	123
5	4	64	127.5
5	5	65	131.5
5	6	66	135.5
5	7	67	139.5
5	8	68	143.5
5	9	69	147.5
5	10	70	151.5

SOURCE: Metropolitan Life Foundation
NOTE: To find ideal weights for adults who fall outside the height ranges shown, consult your physician.

Appendix B
The Stoplight Diet Food Guide

CONTENTS

PROTEIN

YELLOW

Food	Serving Size	Calories
Eggs		
Boiled, hard- or soft-	2 large	160
Omelet, plain	2 large eggs	160
Poached	2 large	160
Scrambled (no fat added)	2 large	160
Sunny-side up (no fat added)	2 large	160
Fish and shellfish (nonfried, unbreaded)		
Anchovies	6 medium	100
Bass	3 ounces	100
Clams	½ cup	100
Cod	3 ounces	100
Crabmeat	½ cup	100
Flounder	3 ounces	100
Haddock	3 ounces	100
Halibut	3 ounces	100
Herring, pickled	1 fillet	100
Lobster	3 ounces	100
Oysters	5 medium	100
Perch	3 ounces	100
Salmon	3 ounces	100
Sardines	3 small	100
Scallops	3 ounces	100
Scrod	3 ounces	100
Shrimp	3 ounces	100
Sole	3 ounces	100
Tuna (fresh, water-packed, or oil-packed and rinsed)	½ cup	100
Whitefish	3 ounces	100
Poultry (nonfried, skinned, unbreaded)		
Chicken breast	3 ounces	150
Chicken drumstick	2 ounces (including bone)	90
Turkey	3 ounces	150

PROTEIN: Yellow (continued)

Food	Serving Size	Calories
Nuts		
Peanut butter	2 tablespoons	190
Red meat (nonfried lean cuts)		
Beef		
Ground (hamburger)	3 ounces	220
Roast	3 ounces	220
Steak	3 ounces	220
Lamb		
Chop	3 ounces	220
Roast	3 ounces	220
Steak	3 ounces	220
Organs		
Heart	3 ounces	220
Kidney	3 ounces	220
Liver	3 ounces	220
Tongue	3 ounces	220
Pork		
Canadian bacon	3 medium slices	200
Chops	3 ounces	220
Ham	3 ounces	220
Roast	3 ounces	220
Veal		
Chop	3 ounces	220
Cutlet	3 ounces	220
Roast	3 ounces	220
Steak	3 ounces	220
Wiener/hot dog/frank	1	140

RED

Food	Serving Size	Calories
Eggs		
Fried in fat	2 large	200
Scrambled in fat	2 large	200

Food	Serving Size	Calories
Fish and shellfish (breaded, fried)		
Breaded	3 ounces	240
Crab cake	3 ounces	150
Fish sticks	4	200
Fried	3 ounces	240
Tuna, oil-packed and unrinsed	½ cup	170
Luncheon meat		
Bologna	2 slices	150
Salami	2 slices	150
Slim Jim	1	85
Nuts (*see also* Other Foods: Red/Seeds)		
Almonds	8	50
Brazil	4	90
Cashews	6 medium	50
Macadamia	6	100
Mixed	8–12	95
Peanuts	6 (1 tablespoon)	90
Pecans	8 halves	50
Pistachios	30	90
Soybeans	1 ounce	130
Walnuts	4 halves	50
Poultry (no skin)		
Capon	3 ounces	200
Chicken, fried	3 ounces	225
Duck	3 ounces	200
Goose	3 ounces	200
Red meat		
Brisket (beef)	3 ounces	350
Corned beef	3 ounces	300
Corned beef hash	1 cup	400
Creamed beef	1 cup	400
Dried beef	3 ounces	180
Pork		
Bacon	2 slices	120

98 · **Appendix B**

PROTEIN: Red (continued)

Food	*Serving Size*	*Calories*
Bacon bits	2 tablespoons	70
Kielbasa	3 ounces	285
Lean 'N Tasty	3 slices	135
Sausage		
Country	3 ounces	300
Links	3	300

GRAINS

YELLOW

Food	Serving Size	Calories
Breads		
Bagel		
Plain	½	80
Water	½	40
Biscuit	1 (2-inch diameter)	80
Bun (hot dog or hamburger)	½	80
Cracked-wheat	1 slice	80
Croutons	1 cup	80
Crumbs		
Dry	¼ cup	80
Soft	½ cup	80
Dinner roll	1 small	80
English muffin	½	80
French	1 slice	80
Italian	1 slice	80
Rye	1 slice	80
Sticks	5 (7¾-inches long)	80
Tortilla shell	1 (6-inch diameter)	80
White	1 slice	80
Whole-wheat	1 slice	80
Cereals, dry (unsweetened)		
All-Bran	⅓ cup	70
Bran, 100-percent	½ cup	70
Bran Chex	⅔ cup	90
Cheerios	¾ cup	80
Corn Chex	¾ cup	80
Cornflakes	¾ cup	80
Cream of Wheat, unsweetened	½ cup (cooked)	80
Farina	½ cup (cooked)	80

GRAINS: *Yellow* (continued)

Food	Serving Size	Calories
Grape-nuts	¼ cup	110
Oatmeal	½ cup (cooked)	80
Puffed rice	1 cup	50
Puffed wheat	1 cup	50
Rice Chex	¾ cup	80
Rice Krispies	¾ cup	80
Shredded Wheat (with bran)	⅔ cup	110
Special K	¾ cup	80
Wheat Chex	¾ cup	80
Wheaties	¾ cup	80
Crackers		
Cheese Tid-Bits	15	80
Goldfish	15	80
Graham	3 (2½×2½ inches)	80
Matzo	1 piece (2×3 inches)	80
Oyster	20	80
Ritz	5	80
Rye Crisp	4 triple crackers	80
Saltines	6 (2×2 inches)	80
Soda	6 (2×2 inches)	80
Triscuits	4	80
Vegetable Thins	4	80
Wheat Thins	8	80
Zweiback	3 pieces	80
Pasta (boiled, no fat added)		
Macaroni	½ cup (cooked)	80
Spaghetti	½ cup (cooked)	80
Rice (boiled, no fat added)		
Brown	½ cup (cooked)	80
White	½ cup (cooked)	80

RED

Food	Serving Size	Calories
Breads and pastries		
Banana bread	1 slice	135
Cornbread	1 slice (2½× 2½×1⅜ inches)	180
Croissant	1	170
Danish pastry	1 (4½-inch diameter)	275
Date-nut bread	1 slice	180
Doughnuts	1	165
French toast	1 slice	120
Muffin	1 (3-inch diameter)	120
Pancake	2 (4-inch diameter)	120
Shake and Bake	4 tablespoons	80
Stuffing	½ cup	210
Sweet roll	1	175
Toaster pastry	1	205
Waffle		
Homemade (in iron)	1	140
Store-bought, toaster	1 (4×4 inches)	90
Cereals		
Barley	¼ cup	175
Breakfast Bar	1	200
Buc Wheats	¾ cup	120
Cream of Wheat, sweetened	½ cup (cooked)	150
With dry fruit (no milk)	¾ cup	120
Farina, sweetened	½ cup (cooked)	150
Fruit and Fiber	¾ cup	120
Granola	¼ cup	130
Life cereal	¾ cup	120
Oatmeal, sweetened	½ cup (cooked)	150
Raisin Bran	¾ cup	120
Sugar-coated (no milk)	¾ cup	120
Pasta		
Chow mein noodles	1 cup	220
Macaroni with fat added	½ cup (cooked)	120

GRAINS: Red (continued)

Food	Serving Size	Calories
Noodles with fat added	½ cup (cooked)	120
Spaghetti with fat added	½ cup (cooked)	120
Rice		
Brown, fried	½ cup	160
Rice-A-Roni	½ cup	125
White, fried	½ cup	160
Wild, boiled	½ cup	110

FRUITS AND VEGETABLES

GREEN

Food	Serving Size	Calories
Nonstarchy vegetables		
Asparagus	½ cup	20
Beans		
Green	½ cup	20
Italian	½ cup	20
Wax	½ cup	20
Bean sprouts	½ cup	20
Beets, boiled	½ cup	20
Broccoli	½ cup	20
Brussels sprouts	4 (½ cup)	20
Cabbage	1 cup	20
Carrots	½ cup	20
Cauliflower	1 cup	20
Celery	1 cup	20
Collards	½ cup	20
Cucumbers	1 cup	20
Eggplant	½ cup	20
Endive	½ cup	20
Kale	½ cup	20
Lettuce	1 cup	10
Mushrooms	1 cup	20
Okra	½ cup	20
Onions	½ cup	20
Parsley	1 cup	20
Peppers	1 cup	20
Radishes	1 cup	20
Rutabaga	¼ cup	20
Salad, tossed	1 cup	20
Sauerkraut	1 cup	20

FRUITS AND VEGETABLES: Green (continued)

Food	Serving Size	Calories
Spinach	1 cup	20
Squash	½ cup	20
Tomato(es)		
Cooked	½ cup	20
Juice	1 cup	40
Paste	2 tablespoons	20
Puree	¼ cup	20
Raw	1 (about 2-inch diameter)	20
Sauce	¼ cup	20
Vegetable juices		
Tomato	1 cup	40
V-8	1 cup	40

YELLOW

Food	Serving Size	Calories
Fruits		
Apple	1 small	40
Applesauce, unsweetened	½ cup	40
Apricots	2	40
Banana	1 small	80
Blackberries	½ cup	40
Blueberries	½ cup	40
Cantaloupe	¾ cup	40
Casaba	¾ cup	40
Cherries	10	40
Grapefruit	½ cup	40
Grapes	12	40
Honeydew melon	⅛ medium (½ cup)	40
Lemon	1	20
Mango	½ small	40
Nectarine	1 medium	40

Food	Serving Size	Calories
Orange	1 small	40
Papaya	¾ cup	40
Peach	1 medium	40
Pear	1 small	40
Pineapple	½ cup	40
Plums	2	40
Pomegranate	½	40
Raspberries	½ cup	40
Strawberries	¾ cup	40
Tangerine	1 medium	40
Watermelon	1 cup	40
Fruit juices		
Apple	⅓ cup	40
Grapefruit	½ cup	40
Orange	½ cup	40
Orange-grapefruit	½ cup	40
Pineapple	⅓ cup	40
Tangerine	½ cup	40
Starchy vegetables		
Artichokes (no fat added)	1	80
Beans		
Chick-peas (garbanzos)	½ cup	80
Kidney	½ cup	80
Lentils	½ cup	80
Lima	½ cup	80
Navy	½ cup	80
Pinto	½ cup	110
Beets, Harvard or pickled	½ cup	80
Corn		
On the cob	1 small ear	120
Shelled kernels	½ cup	80
Mixed	½ cup	80
Parsnips	½ cup	80
Peas	½ cup	80

FRUITS AND VEGETABLES: Yellow (continued)

Food	Serving Size	Calories
Potatoes (no fat added)		
Baked	1 small	80
Boiled	1 small	80
Mashed	½ cup	80
Pumpkin	½ cup	80
Succotash	½ cup	80

RED

Food	Serving Size	Calories
Fruits		
Avocado	¼	80
Dried		
Dates	5	100
Figs	2	80
Prunes	5	85
Raisins	¼ cup	100
Sugared	½ cup	100
Fruit juices		
Apricot nectar	½ cup	70
Cranberry	½ cup	80
Grape	½ cup	80
Peach nectar	½ cup	70
Pear nectar	½ cup	70
Prune	½ cup	100
Rich vegetables (very starchy, creamy, fried)		
Beans		
Baked	½ cup	150
Three-bean salad	½ cup	120
Coleslaw	½ cup	85
Creamed vegetables	½ cup	125

Food	Serving Size	Calories
Potato(es)		
Au gratin	½ cup	130
Baked, with butter	1 small, 1 pat	115
French fries	10 (½ cup)	140
Hash browns	½ cup	180
Mashed, with fat	½ cup	100
Pancakes	1 medium	160
Puffs	½ cup	140
Salad	½ cup	180
Scalloped	½ cup	180
Sweet	½ cup	150
Tater Tots	½ cup	140
Yams (plain)	½ cup	140

DAIRY

YELLOW

Food	Serving Size	Calories
Cheese (skim or low-fat)		
American	1 ounce	100
Blue	1 ounce	100
Brick	1 ounce	100
Cheddar	1 ounce	100
Cottage		
Creamed	½ cup	100
Uncreamed	½ cup	80
Mozzarella	1 ounce	100
Parmesan, grated	3 tablespoons	80
Romano, grated	3 tablespoons	80
Roquefort	1 ounce	100
Swiss	1 ounce	100
Milk (skim or low-fat)		
Buttermilk	1 cup	80
One percent	1 cup	100
Powdered, nonfat	1 cup	80
Skim	1 cup	80
Yogurt (plain)		
Low-fat	½ cup	70
Skim (Colombo)	½ cup	50

RED*

Food	Serving Size	Calories
Ice cream		
Bar, chocolate-covered	1 medium	160
Scooped	½ cup	130
Shake	1 cup	420
Soda	1 cup	260
Soft	½ cup	170
Milk (sweetened, high-fat)		
Chocolate-flavored	1 cup	250
Cocoa/hot chocolate		
Diet	1 cup	70
Regular	1 cup	250
Two percent	1 cup	140
Whole	1 cup	160
Miscellaneous		
Cheese spread	4 tablespoons	160
Eggnog	1 cup	340
Ice milk	½ cup	100
Instant Breakfast	1 cup	280
Pudding		
With skim milk	½ cup	140
With whole milk	½ cup	160
Sherbet	½ cup	130
Yogurt, flavored	½ cup	130

*See also Other Foods: Red/Dairy fats

COMBINATION FOODS

YELLOW*

Food	Serving Size	Calories
Cabbage roll	1 medium	210
Chop suey (with meat but no noodles)	1 cup	300
Chow mein (with no noodles)	1 cup	225
Fish loaf	1 slice (4¹/₈× 2¹/₂×1 inch)	185
Meatloaf	3 ounces	220
Omelet		
Cheese	2 large eggs	260
Vegetable	2 large eggs	260
Pizza, plain	2 5-inch arcs (14-inch diameter)	300
Soup, noncreamy		
Bean	1 cup	90
Beef		
Noodle	1 cup	80
Vegetable	1 cup	80
Chicken		
Gumbo	1 cup	55
Noodle	1 cup	60
Rice	1 cup	50
Vegetable	1 cup	80
Clam chowder, Manhattan	1 cup	80
Onion	1 cup	65
Tomato (with water or skim milk)		
Plain	1 cup	90
Rice	1 cup	110
Turkey		
Noodle	1 cup	80
Vegetable	1 cup	80

*Casseroles, soups, and other combination dishes that contain less than 350 calories per adult serving and no ingredients that are red foods are considered yellow foods.

Food	Serving Size	Calories
Vegetable soup	1 cup	80
Wonton soup	1 cup	90
Spaghetti with plain tomato sauce	1 cup	200
Spanish Rice	1 cup	160
Stew, vegetable-beef	1 cup	220

RED*

Food	Serving Size	Calories
Chicken		
A la king	1 cup	470
Salad	½ cup	280
Chili and beans	1 cup	340
Crab, deviled	1 cup	200
Egg roll	1	300
Egg salad (with mayonnaise)	½ cup	240
Lasagna	1 piece (2×3 inches)	400
Lobster Newburg	½ cup	240
Macaroni and cheese	1 cup	430
Mug-O-Lunch	1 envelope	170
Pot pie	1 small	400
Soups		
Bean with bacon	1 cup	140
Cheese	1 cup	130
Chunky (any variety)	1 cup	170
Clam chowder, New England	1 cup	160
Creamy (any variety)	1 cup	170
Green pea	1 cup	145
Minestrone	1 cup	100
Oyster stew (with milk)	1 cup	130
Split pea	1 cup	145
Tomato (with whole milk)	1 cup	175

*Casseroles, soups, and other combination dishes that contain 350 or more calories per adult serving and those that contain one or more ingredients that are red foods are considered red foods.

COMBINATION FOODS: Red (continued)

Food	Serving Size	Calories
Tuna		
Noodle casserole	1 cup	280
Salad (with mayonnaise)	1 cup	350
Spaghetti with meat sauce	1 cup	330

OTHER FOODS

GREEN

Food	Serving Size	Calories
Condiments and seasonings		
Herbs and spices	any amount	0
Horseradish	any amount	0
Lemon juice	any amount	0
Mustard	any amount	0
Soy sauce	2 tablespoons	0
Vinegar	any amount	0
Worcestershire sauce	any amount	0
Drinks		
Club soda	any amount	0
Coffee, black, unsweetened	any amount	0
Mineral water	any amount	0
Seltzer	any amount	0
Soda pop, diet	any amount	0
Tea, unsweetened	any amount	0
Water	any amount	0
Soups		
Bouillon	1 cup	0
Broth	1 cup	0

YELLOW

Food	Serving Size	Calories
Condiments and seasonings		
A.1. steak sauce	1 tablespoon	20
Barbecue sauce	1 tablespoon	15
Catsup	1 tablespoon	20
Olives		
Black	3	20
Green	4	20

OTHER FOODS: *Yellow* (continued)

Food	Serving Size	Calories
Pickles		
Dill	3 medium	20
Sweet	1 small	22
Relish	1 tablespoon	20
Salad dressing		
French, noncreamy	1 tablespoon	65
Italian, noncreamy	1 tablespoon	80
Oil and vinegar	1 tablespoon	65
Snacks		
Popcorn without butter		
Air-popped	1 cup	20
Popped with oil (2 tablespoons)	1 cup	40
Pretzels		
Dutch	1	60
Rods	1	55
Round	8	60
Three-ring	3	60
Veri-Thin sticks	20	50
Rice cakes	1 large	35

RED

Food	Serving Size	Calories
Cake		
Angelfood (no icing)	1 piece (2×3 inches)	140
With icing	1 piece (2×3 inches)	360
Without icing	1 piece (2×3 inches)	200
Cream puff	1	300
Cupcake (with icing)	1 medium	170
Eclair	1	240
Fruitcake	1 small slice	120
Gingerbread	1 small portion	175
Hostess cake	1	240

Food	Serving Size	Calories
Candy, cookies, and nonfrozen confections		
Animal crackers	10	110
Brownie	1 piece (2×2 inches)	97
Caramel, plain	3 pieces (1 ounce)	115
Chocolate	1 ounce	145
Fudge	1 ounce	115
Gingersnaps	2 (about 2-inch diameter)	60
Gumdrops	5	100
Hard candy	6 pieces	110
Jelly beans	10	104
Lollipop	1 (1 ounce)	110
Marshmallows	3	75
Mints, cream	8	60
Peanut brittle	1 ounce	120
Vanilla wafers	4	75
Dairy fats (*see also* Dairy: Red)		
Butter. *See* Other Foods: Red/Fats and oils		
Cream		
Half and half	2 tablespoons	40
Heavy	1 tablespoon	50
Light	2 tablespoons	60
Whipped	1 tablespoon	25
Cream cheese		
Low-calorie	2 tablespoons	70
Regular	2 tablespoons	100
Margarine. *See* Other Foods: Red/Fats and oils		
Nondairy creamer	1 tablespoon	30
Sour cream	2 tablespoons	50
Drinks		
Alcoholic		
Ale	8 ounces	100
Beer		
Lite	12 ounces	95
Regular	8 ounces	115

OTHER FOODS: *Red* (continued)

Food	Serving Size	Calories
Cordials	1 cordial glass	65
Daiquiri	3½ ounces	120
Gin	1½ ounces	120
Manhattan	3½ ounces	165
Martini	3½ ounces	140
Rum	1½ ounces	120
Vodka	1½ ounces	120
Whiskey		
Shot	1½ ounces	120
Sour	2½ ounces	140
Wine		
Sweet	1 wineglass	140
Table	1 wineglass	85
Nonalcoholic		
Hawaiian Punch	1 cup	120
Hi-C	1 cup	120
Kool-Aid	1 cup	100
Lemonade	1 cup	120
Orangeade	1 cup	120
Quinine water	8 ounces	75
Soda pop		
Large	12 ounces (1½ cups)	145
Small	8 ounces (1 cup)	95
Tang	1 cup	130
Tea, canned, sweetened	12 ounces (1½ cups)	145
Tonic water	8 ounces	90
Fats and oils		
Butter	1 teaspoon	40
Butter Buds	1 tablespoon	6
Margarine		
Diet	1 teaspoon	20
Regular	1 teaspoon	40
Oil (most types)	2 teaspoons	80

Food	Serving Size	Calories
Frozen confections		
(*see also* Dairy: Red)		
Fudgsicle	1	90
Kool Pop	1	30
Popsicle	1	65
Jell-O		
With fruit	½ cup	80
Plain	½ cup	70
Pies		
Custard (1 crust)	⅛ of 9-inch-diameter pie	250
Fruit (all types; 2 crusts)	⅛ of 9-inch-diameter pie	300
Lemon meringue (1 crust)	⅛ of 9-inch-diameter pie	270
Salad dressing		
Blue cheese	1 tablespoon	75
Mayonnaise	1 tablespoon	100
Russian	1 tablespoon	75
Thousand Island	1 tablespoon	80
Sauces		
Butterscotch	2 tablespoons	200
Cheese	¼ cup	105
Chocolate	2 tablespoons	100
Cranberry	2 tablespoons	50
Cream	¼ cup	105
Custard	¼ cup	85
Gravy	2 tablespoons	80
Hollandaise	¼ cup	180
Hot fudge	2 tablespoons	120
Tartar	1 tablespoon	100
Seeds (*see also* Protein: Red/Nuts)		
Pumpkin	3 tablespoons	150
Sesame	3 tablespoons	150
Sunflower	3 tablespoons	150
Snacks		
Bacon rinds	10 rinds (1 ounce)	150
Cheese twists	20 pieces (1 ounce)	160
Corn chips	1 ounce	160
Cracker Jack	1 cup	135
Popcorn with butter	1 cup	140

OTHER FOODS: *Red* (continued)

Food	Serving Size	Calories
Potato		
Chips	1 ounce	160
Sticks	1 cup	196
Sugars and syrups		
Apple butter	1 tablespoon	55
Brown sugar	1 tablespoon	35
Corn syrup	1 tablespoon	60
Honey	1 tablespoon	65
Jam	1 tablespoon	55
Jelly	1 tablespoon	55
Maple		
Sugar	1 ounce	100
Syrup	1 tablespoon	60
Marmalade	1 tablespoon	55
Molasses	1 tablespoon	50
White sugar (granulated or powdered)	1 tablespoon	50

FAST FOODS

YELLOW

Food	Serving Size	Calories
Protein		
Egg, scrambled	1 large	160
Ponderosa		
Prime Rib	4.2 ounces	308
Sirloin Tips	4.0 ounces	293
T-bone Steak	4.3 ounces	315
Grains		
Bagel (no topping)	1	160
English muffin (no butter or topping)	½	80
Fruits and vegetables		
Fruit juices		
Grapefruit	6 ounces	60
Orange	6 ounces	60
Salads (any combination of green and yellow foods under 350 calories)	—	—
Combination Foods		
Arby's		
Junior Roast Beef sandwich	1	220
Roast Beef sandwich	1	350
Cheeseburger, single (except Wendy's)	1	310
Hamburger, single (except Wendy's)	1	260
Pizza Hut cheese pizza	2 slices (13-inch diameter)	340

RED

Food	Serving Size	Calories
Protein		
Arthur Treacher's Fish	2 pieces	340
Long John Silver's		
Chicken Planks	4 pieces	165
Fish	2 pieces	365

FAST FOODS: *Red* (continued)

Food	Serving Size	Calories
McDonald's pork sausage	1 serving	235
Ponderosa		
Imperial Prime Rib	8.4 ounces	616
King Prime Rib	6.0 ounces	439
New York Strip	6.1 ounces	447
Super Sirloin	6.5 ounces	476
Combination Foods		
Arby's		
Beef and Cheese sandwich	1	450
Club sandwich	1	560
Ham and Cheese sandwich	1	380
Super Roast Beef sandwich	1	620
Turkey Deluxe sandwich	1	510
Turkey sandwich	1	410
Burger King		
Chicken sandwich	1	690
Fish sandwich	1	540
Whopper	1	640
Whopper, Jr.	1	280
Long John Silver's		
Fish Sandwich	1	340
McDonald's		
Big Mac	1	560
Chicken McNuggets	6 pieces	225
Egg McMuffin	1	310
Filet-O-Fish	1	400
Double Hamburger	1	350
Half Pounder	1	420
Half Pounder with Cheese	1	520
Quarter Pounder	1	420
Quarter Pounder with Cheese	1	520
Pizza Hut		
Pepperoni pizza	2 slices	370
Superstyle Crispy cheese pizza	2 slices	410
Superstyle pepperoni pizza	2 slices	430

Food	Serving Size	Calories
Other Foods		
Arthur Treacher's		
Chips	1 serving	275
Cole slaw	1 serving	120
Baskin Robbins		
Ice cream (all flavors)	1 scoop	140
Sherbets (all flavors)	1 scoop	140
Burger King		
French fries	1 small serving	240
Shake	1	300
Dairy Queen		
Buster Bar	1	380
Dilly Bar	1	240
Dipped cone	1 large	440
Ice-cream cone	1 large	320
Ice-cream sandwich	1	180
Malt	1 small	400
Parfait	1	400
Sundaes	1 large	420
Dunkin' Donuts		
Donut		
Filled	1	285
Unfilled	1	240
Munchkins		
Plain	6	156
Filled or with toppings	6	246
Long John Silver's		
Hush Puppies	3	150
McDonald's		
Apple pie	1	260
French fries	1 serving	200
Shakes	1	320

Appendix C: Daily Food Chart

Name _____   Date _____

Time	Food or Drink	Amount	Number of Calories	Food Group Color	Basic Four Food Group			
					P	G	F&V	D
Totals								
Goals					2	4	4	3

Appendix D: Daily Weight Chart

Name _____ Week Number ___

Goal Weight _____

Date

	Monday	Tuesday	Wednesday	Thursday	Friday	Saturday	Sunday
	( )	( )	( )	( )	( )	( )	( )

Weight Range (in pounds)

Daily Weight (in pounds)

223

Appendix E: Basic Four Food Group Nutritional Guidelines

Food Group	Recommended Number of Servings per Day	Size of Serving	Primary Nutrients	Main Sources of Primary Nutrients
Protein (P)	2	2 ounces	Protein Iron Niacin Thiamine	Red meat Fish/seafood Poultry Eggs Nuts
Grains (G)	4	1 slice of bread, ½–¾ cup of cereal, or ½ cup of cooked rice or pasta	B vitamins Fiber Vitamin E Iron Protein	Whole grain or enriched products: Bread Cereal Pasta Crackers Rice
Fruits and Vegetables (F&V)	4	1 small piece of fruit, ½–⅔ cup of vegetables, or ½ cup of juice	Vitamin A B vitamins Fiber Vitamin C	Watermelon Carrots Broccoli Cantaloupe Tomatoes Squash Pumpkin Grapefruit Oranges Lemons Limes Tangerines Strawberries Peppers Potatoes

Food Group	Recommended Number of Servings per Day	Size of Serving	Primary Nutrients	Main Sources of Primary Nutrients
				Raw cabbage
				Greens
Dairy (D)	3	1 cup	Calcium	Milk
			Phosphorus	Cheese
			Protein	Yogurt
			Riboflavin	
			Vitamin A	
			Vitamin D	

Appendix F
Sample Stoplight Diet Menus

To help you select meals from the Basic Four food groups on the Stoplight Diet, we offer these sample menus, which will meet the 1,200-calorie-a-day upper limit we suggest for children trying to lose weight on the Stoplight Diet. Remember that these sample menus are just that — samples — which you can follow closely if you wish or modify for your own family's use.

BREAKFASTS

Food and Serving Size	Number of Calories
⅔ cup Bran Chex	90
½ cup blueberries	40
1 cup skim milk	80
½ cup orange juice	40
Total	*250*
1 egg (scrambled in nonstick pan or boiled)	80
1 slice whole-wheat bread	80
1 cup skim milk	80
½ cup orange juice	40
Total	*280*
½ cup oatmeal	80
1 cup skim milk	80
½ cup orange juice	40
Total	*200*

LUNCHES

Food and Serving Size	Number of Calories
2 slices whole-wheat bread	160
2 ounces turkey	100
lettuce and tomato for sandwich	10
1 cup skim milk	80
1 small apple	40
	Total 390

mix together:

2 ounces cooked, diced chicken	100
½ cup chopped celery	10
½ cup low-fat yogurt	70
1 teaspoon curry powder (or to taste)	0

serve on:

1 small whole-wheat pita bread pouch	160
1 small orange	40
	Total 380

mix together:

½ cup rinsed tuna	100
½ cup chopped celery, tomatoes, and carrots	10

serve on:

2 slices whole-wheat bread	160
1 cup skim milk	80
1 medium tangerine	40
	Total 390

DINNERS

Food and Serving Size	Number of Calories
2 ounces baked chicken breast (no skin)	100
½ cup broccoli (with lemon)	20
½ cup cooked rice	80
1 cup tossed salad (lettuce, tomatoes, celery, onions)	20
1 tablespoon oil-and-vinegar salad dressing with herbs	65
½ cup plain skim milk yogurt	40
½ cup fruit	40
	Total 365
2 ounces fillet of sole (broiled, baked, or poached)	67
1 small baked potato	80
1 cup tossed salad (endive, spinach, watercress)	20
1 tablespoon regular Italian salad dressing	80
1 cup skim milk	80
	Total 327
2 slices plain pizza (no meat)	300
1 cup tossed salad	20
1 tablespoon oil-and-vinegar salad dressing	65
1 cup skim milk	80
	Total 465

Appendix G
The Stoplight Diet Contract

_____
date

I, _____, agree to provide _____
    parent's name   *child's name*

with the reward named below once the following conditions are met.

_____ will _____
    child's name   *fill in requirement*

_____

_____

during the next _____. When _____
                time period   *child's name*

has successfully done this, I will provide _____
                                     fill in specific reward

_____

_____.

_____   _____
    parent's signature   *child's signature*

Appendix H

The Stoplight Diet Exercise Guide

CALORIES BURNED DURING TEN MINUTES
OF CONTINUOUS ACTIVITY

Type of Exercise	Body Weight (in pounds)								
	50	*75*	*100*	*125*	*150*	*175*	*200*	*225*	*250*
Walking (2 mph)	12	18	23	30	35	40	46	53	58
Walking (4½ mph)	23	34	45	56	67	78	87	98	110
Walking up stairs	57	88	115	143	175	201	229	259	288
Walking down stairs	23	34	45	56	67	78	88	100	111
Jogging (5½ mph)	36	54	71	90	108	127	142	160	178
Running in place (140 counts/minute)	80	121	163	203	242	284	325	363	405
Bicycling (5½ mph)	12	25	34	42	50	58	67	75	83
Badminton/volleyball	19	28	38	45	52	67	75	85	94
Baseball (not pitcher)	16	24	31	39	47	54	62	70	78
Basketball	23	35	47	58	70	82	93	105	117
Bowling	23	34	45	55	67	82	90	100	111
Dancing (moderate)	14	21	28	34	42	49	55	62	69
Dancing (vigorous)	19	28	38	47	57	67	75	86	94
Square dancing	23	34	45	56	68	80	90	103	113
Football	28	41	55	69	83	97	110	123	137
Golf (foursome)	14	20	28	34	40	47	55	62	68
Horseback riding (trot)	23	34	37	46	67	78	90	102	112
Ping-Pong	13	20	26	32	38	43	52	58	64
Skiing (downhill)	32	48	64	80	96	113	128	145	160
Skiing (cross-country)	40	59	79	99	117	137	158	174	194
Swimming (backstroke; 20 yd/min)	13	20	26	32	38	43	52	58	64
Swimming (breaststroke; 20 yd/min)	16	24	32	40	48	55	63	72	80

SOURCE: Adapted from J. M. Ferguson, *Habits, Not Diets* (Palo Alto, Calif.: Bull Publishing, 1976), 204.

NOTE: Round off the subject's body weight to the closest body weight shown.

Type of Exercise	Body Weight (in pounds)								
	50	75	100	125	150	175	200	225	250
Swimming (crawl; 20 yd/min)	16	24	32	40	48	55	63	72	80
Tennis	23	34	46	58	67	80	92	103	115
Waterskiing	26	39	52	65	73	92	104	117	130
Wrestling/judo/karate	44	66	88	110	129	150	175	192	213

Appendix I
Daily Exercise Chart

Name _____ Week Number ____

Calorie Goal: _____ per day/_____ per week

Day	Date	Type of Exercise	Time Spent Exercising (in minutes)	Number of Extra Calories Burned
Monday				
Tuesday				
Wednesday				
Thursday				
Friday				
Saturday				
Sunday				
			Total	